# The Beating Code: Advancing Cardiac Modeling with Computational Mechanics

Sharlin

First Printing, 2024

# Contents

# 1

# Introduction

The field of computational mechanics has developed considerably over recent decades due to advances in its theoretical formulations and faster, more powerful computational hardware. The use of computational mechanics in research and industry for science/engineering problems is now commonplace, as it has the potential to be a tool of analysis for any variety of solid or fluid mechanics problem. The exciting reality is that current capabilities in computational mechanics only really scratch the surface of truly replicating the near infinite detail of a given physical system. In the quest to advance our capabilities in computational mechanics, there is an on-going iterative progression between the discovery of new enriched mathematical methods to approximate the mechanics of a system, and awaiting adequate computational technology to compute such complex models in a meaningful time frame.

Biological materials and biomechanical processes are often more complex to describe with computational mechanics than conventional inanimate engineering materials. However, the motivations for modelling biomechanics are numerous. Cardiovascular disease is a major cause of global mortality [55], with a World Health Organization (WHO) study ranking it highest at 12.2% [9]. Clearly, there is strong motivation to maximize research into treatments of cardiovascular disease. In turn, the research area of computational cardiac mechanics is expanding rapidly, and brings inter-disciplinary expertise together to bridge the understanding of physiological and mechanical phenomena of the heart.

Clinical treatments have developed over time largely by trial and error, and the testing of new ideas has been stymied by the obvious risks associated with experimenting on *in-vivo* hearts. As computational cardiac models improve, remedial medications and procedures on defective hearts could be prototyped through computational simulations, which are risk-free, cheaper to implement, and faster to adapt and retest. This study will explore the merits of the micromorphic continuum material model to replicate the passive mechanics of the human left ventricle, in order to evaluate on its potential to contribute to cardiac modelling in future.

## 1.1 Current advancements in cardiac modelling

Over the last three decades cardiac modelling has progressed to the point where mathematical models of the complete cardiac cycle are realistic enough to evaluate the performance of the heart and its response to medical treatments. Early cardiac models used rudimentary classical continuum theories that were not able to elucidate the internal structure of the material, and were also limited by basic geometric representations of the heart. Over time so-called multiscale mathematical models have evolved, which begin to incorporate the internal architecture of a material. Additionally, advancements in sophisticated imaging techniques such as electron microscopy, magnetic resonance imaging (MRI) and optimized Diffusion Tensor Imaging (DTI), have expanded physiological knowledge of cardiac (myocardial) tissue [3, 43].

Living tissues constantly morph and adapt through variations in mass and geometry (growth), rearrangement of the micro-structure (remodeling) and shape (morphogenesis) [31]. The long-term objective of cardiac mechanics would be to exhaustively incorporate the myriad physiological, chemical, electrical and mechanical processes of the heart. The orientation of muscle fibres (myocytes) in the heart is a key feature of cardiac tissue and has come under particular focus, as the orientation of myocytes affects not only the passive response of the heart but also its contraction. It has been found in numerous studies that muscle fibre orientation plays a significant role in circumferential and circumferential-radial shear strains in the heart [86, 69]. There remains a lack of experimental data on cardiac tissue, though studies on porcine [12] and human [81] cardiac tissue have shown that the tissue behaves nonlinearly, and further responds differently depending along which direction the material was deformed.

A noteworthy improvement in the mathematics to describe biological tissue behaviour came with the advent of the *Fung*-type strain energy functions through the works of [22, 4, 40]. The *Fung*-type constitutive law is advantageous as it can capture the non-linear stiffness response exhibited by cardiac tissue, and was later expanded upon to include invariant-based models and the fibre-orientated anisotropy that is common to mammalian heart tissue. Furthermore, orthotropic versions of the material law have the flexibility to assign unique stiffness properties to the three characteristic directions of cardiac tissue: the muscle fibres, the banded sheets formed by the muscle fibres, and the direction normal to those sheets. Non-linear orthotropy has been successfully validated in studies such as Usyk et al. (2002) modelling canine left ventricles [87, 88], as well as Holzapfel and Ogden (2009) reproducing shear experiments on porcine ventricular tissue. There are other notable cardiac tissue models, such as Kerckhoffs et al. (2003) and Costa et al. (2001), amongst others.

The improving realism of the mathematical models, coupled with patient-specific heart geometry and data, has enabled cardiac modelling to cultivate remedial work, such as the study of Legner et al. (2014) in analyzing the effect of hydrogel injections into regions of the heart damaged by myocardial infarction. Real-time modelling techniques, such as the work of Rama et al. (2016) on proper orthogonal decomposition with interpolation (PODI), are gaining traction and aim to drastically reduce simulation time by interpolating results from a database of cardiac models [67, 65, 66]. Evidently, great progress has been made in the field of cardiac mechanics; however, there is still tremendous scope for improvement, and it is believed that the micromorphic model explored in this study could become a useful tool in cardiac modelling in future.

## 1.2 Multiscale modelling and micromorphic continuum theory

Continuum models are now widely used to simulate the deformation and failure modes of materials; however, these models rely on averaging of atomic scale dynamics, and subsequently the precision of the models will always be limited if behaviour averaging is employed [50]. Classical continuum models use a representative volume element (RVE) that is large enough to approximate all micro-constituents of the material into an averaged set of material parameters, and therefore nanoscale and molecular processes cannot be described within a continuum mechanics framework. Instead, molecular dynamics (MD) models can be used for such intricate simulations; however, the computational cost of MD models render them impractical for use on common engineering problems. The so-called multiscale models, named for their ability to account for some of the micro-architecture of a material, are still based on continuum theory, and although they use some simple statistical averaging, they are not founded on molecular theories nor statistical mechanics [16]. Multiscale models are the most effective models in use today, because they give a richer description of a material's structure and composition over classical continuum models, whilst completing simulations in a relevant time frame.

Various multiscale models evolved during the 20th century. Noteworthy generalized continuum theories include Cosserat theory devised by the Cosserat brothers [Cosserat and Cosserat (1909)], microstructure theory [Mindlin (1964)], micromorphic theory [Eringen and Suhubi (1964)], and micropolar theory [Eringen (1966)]. More recently the FE2 multilevel finite element method, such as Geers et al. (2007) and Schröder (2014), has emerged as an exciting form of multiscale modelling, which includes a separate micro-simulation to homogenize micro-scale properties with greater detail of the micro-structure. However, the drawback of using the FE2 method is in its computational overhead. An example of multiscale modelling is that of granular materials, where the size and properties of the individual granular particles and the orientations of the granules can be incorporated [54]. Available studies on cardiac tissue mechanics using generalized continuum models include the use of one-dimensional Cosserat continua by Sack et al. (2016), and a micromorphic medium by Thurieau et al. (2017), amongst others.

This research explores the micromorphic theory which caters for the local micro-structure and intrinsic motions of the material. Eringen (1966) believed the theory showed great promise for tackling many phenomena, that were previously poorly modelled using a statistical mechanics approach. The micromorphic theory offers the flexibility to encompass surface tension, couple stress, inertial spin, distributed vortices and micro-anisotropy. However, Eringen did concede that the efficacy and success of the model would need to be determined through future experimentation, and as such the author intends to assess its suitability to cardiac modelling.

A micromorphic material contains a collection of deformable vectors, referred to as micro-directors. In the context of cardiac mechanics, the micro-directors can represent muscle fibres and capture non-affine deformations of the muscle fibres relative to the tissue surrounding them. This research utilizes the novel interpretation of the micromorphic theory developed by Sansour (1998), Sansour and Skatulla (2009), Sansour et al. (2010) and von Hoegen et al. (2017), which attempts to overcome shortfalls in Eringen's strain measures in terms of Euler-Lagrange equations by supplementing new strain measures and corresponding field equations [73].

## 1.3 Motivation, aim and objectives

Numerical models are already used as a non-invasive technique to test new treatment ideas regarding surgery and pharmacology for the heart. This includes prototyping mechanical alterations to the cardiac system, such as the use of hydrogels to treat infarcted heart tissue [51], or looking at the impact of rotary blood pumps on heart function [58]. However, the detail and precision of mathematical models are still limited by crude approximations of cardiac tissue and its behaviour. Currently muscle fibre reorientation for classical models has been dealt with algorithmically or with additional iterative procedures such as that done generally by Himpel et al. (2008), Hariton et al. (2006) and Fausten et al. (2016) who modelled collagen fibre reorientation in arterial walls. In such algorithmic schemes, a preferred fibre direction is consecutively identified based on the principal tensile stresses caused by a specific loading condition, and subsequently the stress is recalculated for the new adjusted preferred fibre direction.

The micromorphic model will be used to replicate the motion of muscle fibres without the need for computationally expensive and algorithmically treated procedures. The implementation of the model will be done in *SESKA* (see Appendix B), which is the in-house modelling software used .by the Computational Continuum Mechanics (CCM) group at the University of Cape Town. This study continues from the work of von Hoegen et al. (2016) where a micromorphic model was calibrated to porcine cardiac tissue shear experiments, and will calibrate a similar micromorphic model to human cardiac tissue shear experiments. Numerical artifacts of Sansour's generalized micromorphic model are assessed to better understand the mechanisms driving the model, and novel proofs are devised by the author. The author's own alternative MDO micromorphic model is assessed as it attempts to counteract potential numerical artifacts of Sansour's micromorphic model that were uncovered in this study.

Cardiovascular disease is a top cause of global morality [55], and therefore cardiac research is of great importance. Furthermore, the left ventricle is most susceptible to myocardial infarctions due to its size and workload, and will therefore be the focal point of this research topic given its importance. This study uses a micromorphic model to simulate the left ventricle using patient-specific data segmented by Hopkins (2017) from 3D cardiac magnetic resonance (CMR) scans of the human heart provided by Cape Universities Body Imaging Centre (CUBIC). Particular focus will be placed on the ability of the micromorphic micro-director to represent myocytes, and the potential for non-affine motion of the myocytes relative to the bulk tissue surrounding them. This study will thus serve as a necessary first step towards applying micromorphic continuum theory to patient-specific cardiac models, with patient-specific modelling likely to be a staple of future medical treatments.

In summary this MSc book has the following aims:

- Assess the behaviour of the micromorphic model through a variety of numerical examples.
- Analyse the micromorphic model's behaviour in terms of its mathematical formulation and provide corresponding novel proofs.
- Introduce the author's own interpretation of the micromorphic model to avoid undesirable numerical artifacts of Sansour's micromorphic model uncovered in this study.
- Calibrate Sansour's micromorphic model to experimental cardiac data.
- Simulate the passive filling phase of the left ventricle using Sansour's micromorphic model, and assess its ability to account for non-affine motion of myocytes relative to the bulk tissue surrounding them.

## 1.4 Scope and limitations

The micromorphic continuum does offer limited resolution of micro-scale phenomena; however, it is still a gross approximation of the makeup and intricacies of cardiac tissue. The challenge posed by micromorphic theory is that it requires many material constants [97], and the problem therefore arises of how do we correctly measure those constants? Due to lack of experimental data distinguishing the properties of different components of cardiac tissue, this study relies on assumed contributions only. This study will not explore the active mechanics of the cardiac cycle due to scope limitations. Physiological simplifications into a mechanics framework are made, such as replacing the blood filling the ventricular cavity with just a pressure force. It is worth noting that the mechanical behaviour of the heart can be significantly altered by cardiovascular pathologies, such as cardiomyopathy; however, these heart conditions are not examined in this study.

## 1.5 Layout of book

Following this introductory chapter, the physiology of the heart is introduced in Chapter 2, which focuses on the features and processes included in present-day cardiac models, such as muscle fibre composition and orientation. Classical continuum mechanics is discussed in Chapter 3, as it forms the fundamental framework for computational cardiac mechanics. The concepts of kinematics and stress are explained, along with the hyperelastic constitutive laws used to link stress to strain. The micromorphic continuum model used in this study is examined in Chapter 4, including the derivation of its strain measures and variational principles. The numerical examples of Chapter 5 explore simple problems to highlight the characteristics of the micromorphic model, including micro-director displacement, model instabilities, and strain dependent anisotropy. Additionally, the author's own proposed micromorphic model is assessed as it attempts to counteract potential numerical artifacts of Sansour's micromorphic model that were uncovered in this study. The cardiac models investigated during this research are presented in Chapter 6, which includes model calibration to cardiac tissue experiments and models of the passive filling phase of the heart cycle. Finally, a summary of the conclusions made in this study is presented in Chapter 7, and recommendations for future use of micromorphic modelling in cardiac mechanics are provided.

# 2

# Cardiac Mechanics

Scientific understanding of the makeup, composition, and even function of the human heart has come a long way over recent centuries. Interestingly, it was historically believed that the heart's function was to produce heat for the body, and it was not until 1628 that William Harvey concluded that the heart's purpose was to pump blood around the body and that this was reason for the heartbeat [62]. Biological tissue adapts to the mechanical demands of its environment - an example is the loss of bone mass and muscle atrophy caused by weightlessness. Furthermore, living tissue constantly morphs and adapts through variations in mass and geometry (growth), rearrangement of its micro-structure (remodeling) and shape (morphogenesis) [31]. The physiology and mechanics of the heart and its left ventricle are outlined in this section, as these features need to be incorporated into the mathematical model where possible to ensure the relevance of the numerical approximations achieved.

## 2.1 Structure

The heart has four chambers for pumping blood - the left and right atria and the left and right ventricles, as illustrated in Figure 2.1. The atria are smaller and have thinner walls than the ventricles, because the atria only need to pump blood to the adjacent ventricles and thus develop lower pressures. The ventricles are tasked with pumping blood around the body. The right ventricle sends blood through the pulmonary artery to be oxygenated and expel carbon dioxide in the lungs. The left ventricle is the biggest pump in the heart, with almost double the thickness and triple the mass of the right ventricle, as it must generate enough pressure to transport blood through the aorta to service the entire body [44]. The left ventricle is most susceptible to myocardial infarctions due to its size and workload, and will therefore be the focal point of this research topic given its importance.

The heart is predominately comprised of muscle fibres, known as the myocardium, which generate the pumping action through synchronized contractions. The ventricle wall was found to be thickest towards the top of the ventricles, also referred to as the base, where the atria connect to the ventricles [27]. The bottom tip of the heart is referred to as the apex. The heart is encased in a thin sheet of tissue called the pericardium that is mainly composed of collagen. It is so thin that its mechanical properties can be treated as two-dimensional, and because it sits on the outer surface of the heart, it can be excised and tested with limited risk to the patient [21]. The epicardium is a thin layer of tissue on the outer surface of the cardiac tissue, and is adjacent to the pericardium. The cavities of

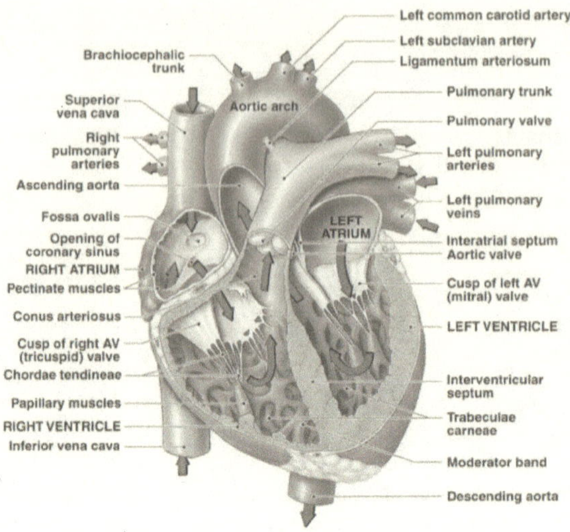


Fig. 2.1: Annotated cross-section of the human heart [95].

the atria and the ventricles are lined by another thin layer of tissue called the endocardium - refer to Figure 2.2.

## 2.2 Myocardium

The heart wall muscle tissue, or myocardium, is predominately composed of muscle cells known as myocytes, which are held together by connective tissue called the extracellular matrix (ECM). The myocytes are long extended cells, typically between $50 - 150\mu m$ in length and $10 - 20\mu m$ in diameter [25], and are grouped together in helical bands that wrap around the heart as shown in Figure 2.5. Probing deeper into the micro-structure of the myocardium we find that myocytes are made up of cross-striated myofibrils, as well as mitochondria which produce the energy required for contraction in the form of phosphates [44], in conjunction with the calcium concentration in the ECM [45]. Further, the myofibrils are divided into sarcomeres, which are a collection of myosin and actin filaments seen in Figure 2.3. The sarcomere length helps govern the contractile force of the muscle, and the working range of sarcomere length is $1.9 - 2.2\mu m$ [26]. The velocity of shortening of the sarcomeres during contraction is also important to maintain the contractile force in the muscle as the activations of contraction are not uniform throughout the heart [11]. It is hoped the micro-director of the micromorphic model, a method of fibre representation, can be suitably used to approximate the behaviour of the myocytes in this study.

Collagen is also the most abundant protein in the ECM; it is also the most common protein in the human body and provides 90% of bone matrix protein content. Collagen serves an important function by maintaining myocyte alignment. The composition of the ECM can be seen clearly in Figure 2.4,

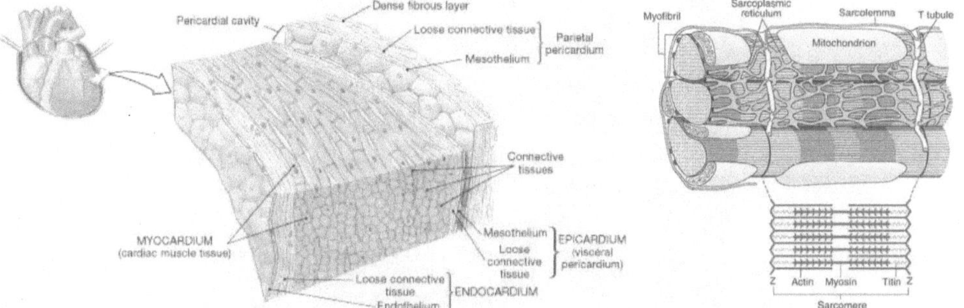


Fig. 2.2: Layers of the heart: the pericardium, epicardium, myocardium, and endocardium [68].

Fig. 2.3: Composition of myocytes [32].

as a result of current advancements in electron microscopy [43]. The connective tissue of the ECM is distinguished by the endomysium surrounding each myocyte, the perimysium supporting groups of myocytes, and the epimysium enveloping the entire muscle. Collagen of the ECM and titin of the cytoskeletal proteins are the most dominant contributors to passive stiffness. Titin mostly accounts for stiffness at smaller strains of the working range and collagen for larger strains. This is further elaborated upon in regards to relevant constitutive law in Section 4.4 and documented in Figure 2.9. The ECM contributions to the mechanics of the heart will be attributed to the macro-scale components of the micromorphic model in this study.

## 2.3 Muscle fibre orientation

The muscle fibres in the left ventricle are joined together to form sheets that span the thickness of the heart wall, and the orientation of the muscle fibres changes across these sheets. The muscle fibres form helical bands with the epicardial fibres arranged in a counterclockwise spiral and the endocardial fibers directed in a clockwise spiral from apex to base [56], as observed in Figure 2.5 and Figure 2.6. It has been found in numerous studies that fibre orientation plays a significant role in circumferential and circumferential-radial shear strains in the heart [86, 69].

In order to model the fibre distribution in the left ventricle, an orthogonal local fibre coordinate system is introduced. The myocyte orientation is represented in Fig(2.7d) with the myocytes *fibre axis* ($\mathbf{V}_f$), the sheets formed by connected myocytes *sheet axis* ($\mathbf{V}_s$), and the axis normal to the sheet *sheet-normal axis* ($\mathbf{V}_n$). The fibre angles were historically extracted *ex vivo*; however, it is now possible to record fibre angles *in vivo* through the use of sophisticated imaging techniques such as magnetic resonance imaging (MRI) and optimized Diffusion Tensor Imaging (DTI) [3].

The transmural variation of muscle fibre angles is illustrated in Fig(2.7c). In the case of canine left ventricles, Streeter et al. (1969) found the endocardium to have a fibre angle of approximately $+60°$ relative to the circumferential direction, and $-60°$ at the epicardium. Wong and Kuhl (2014) used histological studies and DTI to conclude that human left ventricles have fibre angles of approximately

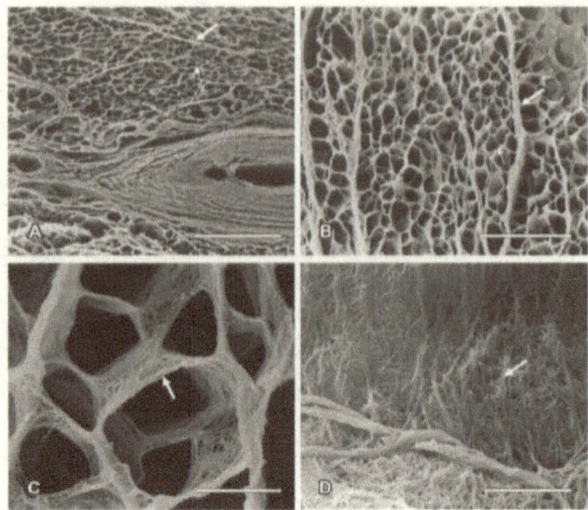


Fig. 2.4: Transverse section of the connective tissue of the human heart. **A)** The collagen network surrounding cardiomyocytes. **B)** The interstitial connective tissue comprised of endomysial and perimysial components presents a honeycomb shape. The perimysium (thick arrow) surrounds groups of cardiomyocytes, and the endomysium (thin arrow) surrounds each cardiomyocyte. **C)** The endomysium holds and joins individual cardiomyocyte fascicles. **D)** At greater magnification collagen fibers exhibit interconnections on the surface of cardiomyocytes. [43].

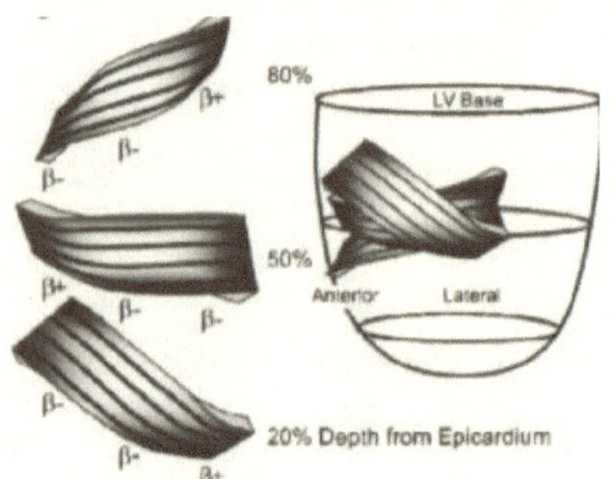


Fig. 2.5: Muscle fibre helical grouping and fibre orientation in the left ventricle [25].

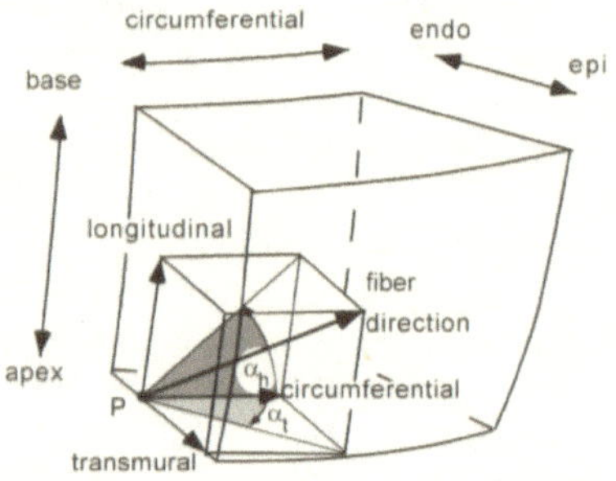

Fig. 2.6: Illustration of the helix ($\alpha_h$) and transverse ($\alpha_t$) fibre angles in a through-wall block of tissue taken from the left ventriclar wall [69].

+80° for the endocardium, and −70° for the epicardium, and Papadacci et al. (2017) found the absolute difference in fibre angle for epicardium to endocardium to be 104° ± 9°. Fibre orientation is not only relevant to the heart's passive mechanics. Roberts et al. (1979) found that cardiac fibre orientation is also important for electrical conduction velocity and tissue resistivity in canine hearts. The direction of the force generated due to muscle contraction is also dependent on muscle fibre orientation, and it is hoped that the micromorphic model will be more effective and versatile than classical models at capturing changes in fibre orientation.

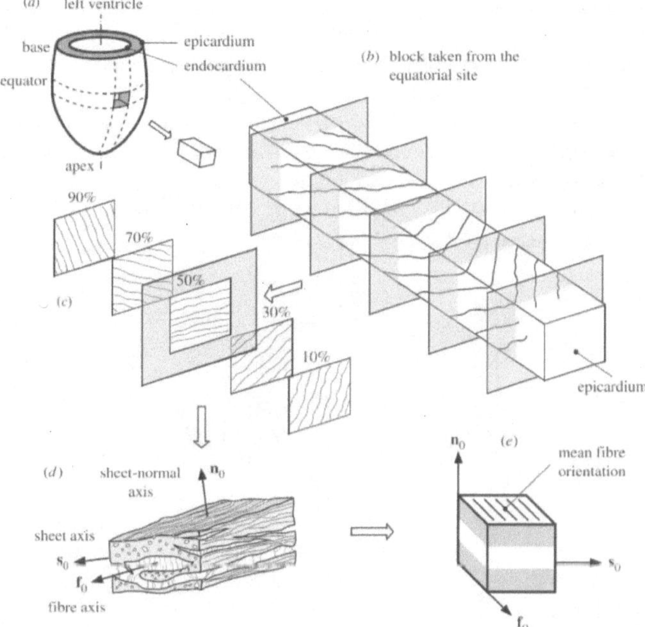


Fig. 2.7: Schematic diagram of: **a)** the left ventricle and a tissue sample from the equator; **b)** the composition through the thickness of the heart wall; **c)** five longitudinal-circumferential sections at uniform intervals from 10% to 90% of the wall thickness from the epicardium showing the transmural variation of fibre orientation; **d)** the layered arrangement of myocytes and the collagen fibres between sheets define an orthogonal local fibre coordinate system $(\mathbf{f}_0, \mathbf{s}_0, \mathbf{n}_0)$; and **e)** idealized cube based on local fibre coordinate system with mean fibre orientation for $\mathbf{f}_0$ [35].

Muscle fibre orientation can be modelled using a prolate spheroid coordinate system, where the radial coordinate is interpolated using Hermite basis functions that preserve continuity [60]. The fibre vectors in the left ventricle were set up using an algorithm developed by Wong and Kuhl (2014) to solve a scalar-valued *Poisson* problem, which is a computationally inexpensive method of fibre vector generation that accounts for the non-uniformity of the ventricular surface. However, the interpolation of the muscle fibre orientation through the heart wall was achieved using the moving least squares based approximation of Skatulla and Sansour (2016), as it is considerably faster than solving the *Poisson* problem, whilst maintaining the helical spiral of the muscles fibres.

## 2.4 Phases of the cardiac cycle

The cardiac cycle, more commonly referred to as the heartbeat, has two phases; the period of muscle contraction is termed systole, and the period after contraction in which the heart relaxes and refills with blood is termed diastole. The systole is divided into two sections: *isovolumetric contraction* where the left ventricle contracts to pressurize the blood but with the aortic valve and mitral valve still closed and thus no volume change in the left ventricular chamber; and *ejection* when the aortic valve opens to let blood pump out through the ascending aorta to the body and the left ventricular volume decreases. The diastole is also split into two sections: *isovolumetric relaxation* as the muscle is still contracted but begins relaxing, before the mitral valve opens to allow blood from the lungs to enter; and *passive filling* as blood refills the left ventricle and the heart wall is relaxed and expands to accommodate the influx of oxygenated blood. These phases of the cardiac cycle and their impact on the ventricular volume, pressure and electrical signal are illustrated in Figure 2.8.

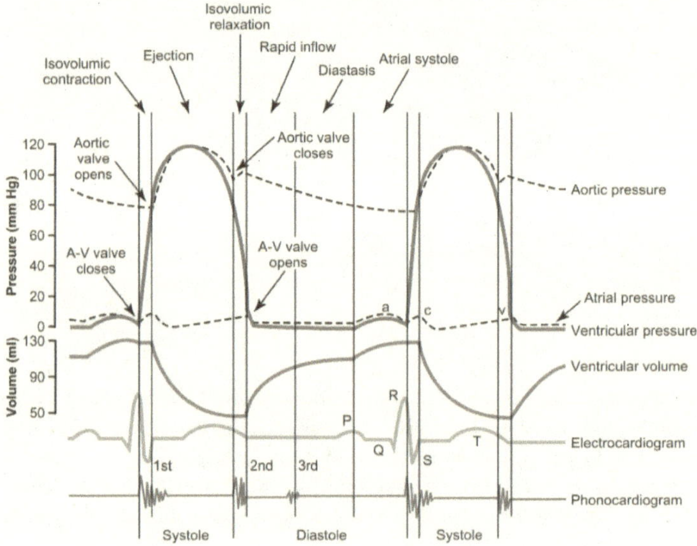


Fig. 2.8: Events of the cardiac cycle for left ventricle function illustrated in a simplified Wiggers diagram. The electrocardiogram exhibits the 'P' wave of atrial depolarization, the 'QRS' waves are ventricular depolarization, and the 'T' wave is ventricular re-polarization. [29].

The Frank-Starling law of the heart states that for an increase in ventricular volume, there is a rise in pressure development or stroke volume. Further, there is myofilament length dependent activation, in which the stretch of the myofilament regulates the contraction activation [45]. Therefore, it is proposed that the micromorphic model micro-director stretching could be coupled with the myofilament length dependent activation in future work. More complex biological phenomena occur after diastolic filling, such as active contraction involving calcium ion concentration, and sophisticated modelling techniques are required to meaningfully mimic the minutia of detail in such phenomena. Modelling further phases of the cardiac cycle after diastolic filling is beyond the scope of this research; however, the reader is referred to examples where other processes of the cardiac cycle are studied [84, 38].

## 2.5 Passive mechanics

Granzier and Irving (1995) performed experiments on rat cardiac tissue and found that collagen and titin are the main contributors to the passive response of the myocardium. The intracellular titin proteins of the muscle fibres were found to account for a large part of the stiffness at short sarcomere lengths, while collagen was found to dominate the stiffness at longer lengths - accounting for about 80% of the total stiffness at a sarcomere length of 2.20 $\mu$m [26]. During diastole the perimysial collagen begins to uncoil under small strains, later becoming fully extended under large strains, which drastically increases the stiffness of the tissue, and protects the myocytes from overstretch. Therefore, the collagen of the ECM accounts for the sharp spike in the pressure-volume curve and the stress-strain curve seen in Figure 2.9(D). In Figure 2.9(A-C) there are two perpendicular orientations of collagen; the perimysial collagen and the collagen struts, which give unique stiffness contributions when strained in their directions, thus motivating the use of non-linear orthotropy to represent the ECM.

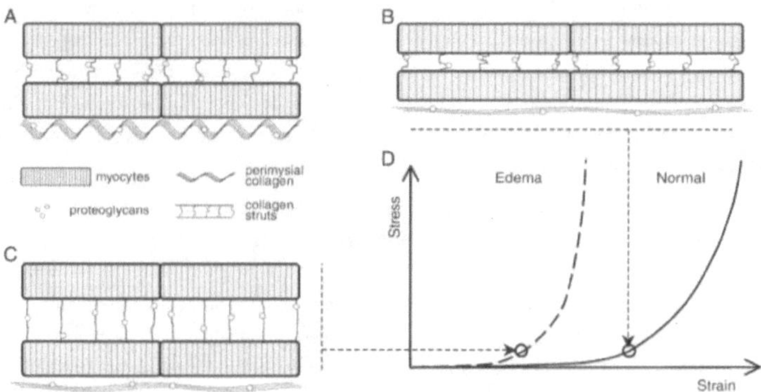


Fig. 2.9: Extracellar matrix (ECM) component contributions to myocardial mechanics. **A)** Diagram displays myocytes connected by collagen struts, perimysial collagen fibers orientated with the myocytes, and proteoglycans associated with the collagen. **B)** Subjected to passive uniaxial stretch, titin in myocytes initially absorbs most of the force as perimysial collagen fibers uncoil; once straightened, collagen resists further extension, protecting myocytes from overstretch. **C)** Both perimysial collagen and collagen struts fully uncoiled. **D)** Increase in resistance seen from prestressed collagen network. [21].

The constitutive law used to describe the passive mechanics is discussed in Section 3.5 for classical mechanics, and in Section 4.4 for micromorphic mechanics. Both the classical constitutive model and macro-scale portion of the micromorphic constitutive model of this study make use of an orthotropic, non-linear constitutive law introduced by Usyk et al. (2002). This study will not explore the active mechanics of the cardiac cycle due to scope limitations. It is worth noting that the mechanical behaviour of the heart can be significantly altered by cardiovascular pathologies, such as cardiomyopathy; however, these heart conditions are also not examined in this study.

# 3

# Classical Continuum Theory

Matter comprises of molecules, which are formed from even smaller particles known as atoms. The behaviour of the molecular components, as well as the other micro-scaled architectures of a material, results in a near infinitely complex material behaviour when subjected to forces. Further to this, when examining a material in minute detail, we find that it is not continuous, because there are voids between its molecular components. However, when modelling common engineering problems, such as the deflection of a structure under loads, the drag force experienced by a plane traveling through air, or for this research topic the filling phase of the human heart, it is possible to describe and predict these gross (macro-scale) phenomena using continuum mechanics without addressing the molecular structure of materials [48].

Continuum mechanics is based on the assumption that a material body is continuous, entirely fills the space it occupies and is indefinitely divisible. We can characterize a material as a continuous medium and approximate a very large number of particles with just a few key field quantities, such as stiffness, density and temperature, which we then consider to be a macroscopic system [34]. Importantly, our choice of a representative macroscopic continuum should try to represent averages over dimensions that are small enough to capture high gradients and incorporate rudimentary micro-structural effects. The topic of continuum mechanics can be divided into the following three areas:

- Kinematics (motion and deformation)
- Stress
- Balance principles (laws of physics)

The term classical continuum mechanics describes the most general form of continuum mechanics that only allows for one degree of freedom per dimension to describe the position and composition of any point in a body. Classical continuum theory has been expanded upon in various ways to produce richer multiscale continuum theories that begin to incorporate the internal architecture of a material on a so-called micro-scale. Such multiscale continuum theories include amongst others: a micropolar continuum, a Cosserat continuum, a microstretch continuum and a micromorphic continuum. This section will outline the fundamentals of the classical continuum theory, which will later be expanded upon in Section 4 to include the micro-scale additions of a micromorphic continuum.

## 3.1 Kinematics of the classical continuum

The kinematics of a body refers to the placement or position of a point within a body, and to where that point deforms or displaces over time due to unbalanced forces acting on the body, without reference to the causal forces. Consider a body $\mathcal{B}$ in a three-dimensional Euclidean vector space in its undeformed or reference configuration, also referred to as the material or Lagrangian description. $\mathcal{B}$ is positioned in space with parameters of generalized coordinates $X_1, X_2$ and $X_3$, which are associated with generalized bases vectors denoted by $\mathbf{G}_1, \mathbf{G}_2$ and $\mathbf{G}_3$, respectively. The most common form of a three-dimensional Euclidean vector space is that of a Cartesian coordinate system, which is orthogonal (all axes are perpendicular).

After subjecting a body to specific boundary conditions, the body at time $t$ is denoted by $\mathcal{B}_t$ in its deformed or current configuration, also known as the spatial or Eulerian description. In order to describe the transformation of the shape of the body, we introduce a non-linear deformation map $\varphi : \mathcal{B} \to \mathcal{B}_t$, which defines the relation of a material point in the undeformed configuration ($\mathbf{X} \in \mathcal{B}$), to that of a unique spatial point in the deformed configuration ($\mathbf{x} \in \mathcal{B}_t$). Conversely, the inverse map $\varphi^{-1} : \mathcal{B}_t \to \mathcal{B}$ returns the deformed material point back to its undeformed position

$$\mathbf{x} = \varphi\left(\mathbf{X}, t\right), \quad \text{and} \quad \mathbf{X} = \varphi^{-1}\left(\mathbf{x}, t\right). \tag{3.1}$$

The gradient and divergence operators with respect to the undeformed (material) configuration and the deformed (spatial) configuration are considered in Table 3.1.

Table 3.1: Gradient and divergence operations in the material and spacial configurations.

| Operator | Reference Configuration | Deformed Configuration |
|---|---|---|
| Gradient | $Grad(\bullet) = \frac{\partial}{\partial \mathbf{X}}(\bullet) = \boldsymbol{\nabla}(\bullet)$ | $grad(\bullet) = \frac{\partial}{\partial \mathbf{x}}(\bullet) = \boldsymbol{\nabla}_t(\bullet)$ |
| Divergence | $Div(\bullet) = \frac{\partial}{\partial X_i}(\bullet) \cdot \mathbf{e}_i = \boldsymbol{\nabla} \cdot (\bullet)$ | $div(\bullet) = \frac{\partial}{\partial x_i}(\bullet) \cdot \mathbf{e}_i = \boldsymbol{\nabla}_t \cdot (\bullet)$ |

The deformation gradient, $\mathbf{F}$, is found from the gradient of $\varphi$. The displacement field is defined as $\mathbf{u}(\mathbf{X}, t) = \mathbf{x}(\mathbf{X}, t) - \mathbf{X}$, and thus $\mathbf{F}$ can be alternatively formulated in terms of $\mathbf{u}(\mathbf{X}, t)$

$$\mathbf{F} := \frac{\partial \boldsymbol{x}}{\partial \boldsymbol{X}} = Grad(\varphi) = \mathbf{I} + \boldsymbol{\nabla}\mathbf{u} \tag{3.2}$$

The following summarized relations are all useful for mapping different geometric properties from a material configuration to its spatial configuration. We map line elements of a material configuration $d\mathbf{X}$ to its corresponding spatial configuration $d\mathbf{x}$ using the deformation gradient,

$$d\mathbf{x} = \mathbf{F}d\mathbf{X}. \tag{3.3}$$

The *Jacobian* $J$ is calculated as the determinant of $\mathbf{F}$, and is used to help map area and volume elements

$$J = det\mathbf{F} = det(Grad\varphi). \tag{3.4}$$

We map area elements using Nanson's formula; it relates the surface element in its reference configuration $dA$, with unit normal $\mathbf{n}$, to its respective surface element in the spatial configuration $da$, with unit normal $\boldsymbol{\nu}$, by

$$\boldsymbol{\nu} da = J\,\mathbf{F}^{-T}\mathbf{n}\, dA. \tag{3.5}$$

Finally, we map the volume change a body undergoes from $\mathcal{B}$ to $\mathcal{B}_t$ using $J$. We note that $J$ must be positive, as a material can be compressed but cannot disappear. Also we find that $J = 1$ for an incompressible material, or if the motion of the body is volume preserving (isochoric motion).

$$dv = JdV \tag{3.6}$$

The deformation gradient is a proper measure of strain; however, it contains rotations that are irrelevant when determining the deformation of a material. Therefore, we seek strain measures that capture the relative deformation of a material. To do this we first calculate the quadratic stretch in the length of a line after deformation from the spatial configuration $d\mathbf{x}^2$, to the material configuration $d\mathbf{X}^2$, as follows

$$d\mathbf{x} \cdot d\mathbf{x} = \mathbf{F}d\mathbf{X} \cdot \mathbf{F}d\mathbf{X} = d\mathbf{X} \cdot (\underbrace{\mathbf{F}^T\mathbf{F}}_{\mathbf{C}})d\mathbf{X}, \tag{3.7}$$

whereby the right *Cauchy-Green* deformation tensor $\mathbf{C}$ is defined as

$$\mathbf{C} = \mathbf{F}^T\mathbf{F}. \tag{3.8}$$

From here we derive the *Green-Lagrange strain tensor* $\mathbf{E}$, which represents the changes of lengths in the continuum due to the displacements of the material points:

$$\mathbf{E} = \frac{1}{2}(\mathbf{C} - \mathbf{I}) = \frac{1}{2}\left(\mathbf{F}^T\mathbf{F} - \mathbf{I}\right). \tag{3.9}$$

## 3.2 Classical stress measures

A body subjected to external forces will deform in response to those forces and develop a distribution of internal forces that are referred to as stresses. External forces acting on a body $\mathcal{B}$ are categorized by body forces $\mathbf{b}$ applied to the entire material, such as gravity, or by surface tractions $\mathbf{t}^{(\boldsymbol{\nu})}$ acting on a material surface with unit normal $\boldsymbol{\nu}$, such as pressure. For the resulting force $\Delta\mathbf{f}$ acting on a surface $\Delta a$ within the body $\mathcal{B}_t$, the *Cauchy stress* principle produces the traction vector $\mathbf{t}^{(\boldsymbol{\nu})}$ with unit normal $\boldsymbol{\nu}$:

$$\lim_{a\to 0} \frac{\Delta\mathbf{f}}{\Delta a} = \frac{\partial\mathbf{f}}{\partial a} = \mathbf{t}^{(\boldsymbol{\nu})}. \tag{3.10}$$

The stress state at any point in the deformed body $\mathbf{x} \in \mathcal{B}_t$ is calculated as follows

$$\mathbf{t}^{(\boldsymbol{\nu})}(\mathbf{x}, t) = \boldsymbol{\sigma}^T(\mathbf{x}, t)\,\boldsymbol{\nu}(\mathbf{x}, t), \tag{3.11}$$

where the axial and shear stresses at a particular deformed point $\mathbf{x}$ are contained in the *Cauchy stress* tensor $\boldsymbol{\sigma}$. Conversely, if the stress is desired for the same particular point but with respect to its undeformed configuration with surface $dA$, and undeformed unit normal $\mathbf{n}$, then the *Cauchy stress lemma* of Eq. (3.10) becomes

$$\mathbf{t}^{(\mathbf{n})}(\mathbf{X}, t) = \boldsymbol{P}^T(\mathbf{X}, t)\,\boldsymbol{n}(\mathbf{X}, t), \tag{3.12}$$

where $\boldsymbol{P}$ is the first *Piola-Kirchhoff* stress tensor, which is instead a function of $\mathbf{X}$. It is beneficial to define yet another stress measure, the second *Piola-Kirchhoff* $\mathbf{S}$, which is fully expressed in the undeformed configuration, and is related to $\mathbf{P}$:

$$\mathbf{P} = \mathbf{FS}. \tag{3.13}$$

Furthermore, if we assume that a force acting on $d\mathbf{a}$ is no different from the force acting on $d\mathbf{A}$, then

$$d\mathbf{f} = \mathbf{Pn}\,dA = \boldsymbol{\sigma}^T\boldsymbol{\nu}\,da = \boldsymbol{\sigma}^T det(\mathbf{F})\mathbf{F}^{-T}\mathbf{n}\,dA. \tag{3.14}$$

Finally we can reformulate the first *Piola-Kirchhoff* as

$$\mathbf{P} = det\,(\mathbf{F})\,\boldsymbol{\sigma}^T\mathbf{F}^{-T} \tag{3.15}$$

## 3.3 Balance laws of continuum mechanics

Continuum mechanics is underpinned by the fundamental laws of physics and consequently any change to a property in a system, such as force or temperature, must abide by these laws. A summary of the three influential laws is listed here:

- **Conservation of mass:** The mass of a system is conserved and hence the change of mass must be zero. Therefore an infinitesimal mass element in the undeformed and deformed configurations must be equal.

$$m = \int_{\mathcal{B}_t} \rho\,(\mathbf{x}, t)\;dv = \int_{\mathcal{B}} \rho_0\,(\mathbf{X})\;dV \tag{3.16}$$

- **Conservation of linear and angular momentum:** The principle of the balance of linear momentum states that the change in linear momentum in time is equal to the sum of all external forces acting on the volume and surfaces of a body $\mathcal{B}$ [94]:

$$\int_{\mathcal{B}_t} \rho\,(\mathbf{x}, t)\,\mathbf{a}\,dv = \int_{\partial\mathcal{B}_t} \mathbf{t}^{(\nu)}\,(\mathbf{x}, t)\;da + \int_{\mathcal{B}_t} \mathbf{b}\,(\mathbf{x}, t)\;dv. \tag{3.17}$$

  By making use of the *Gauss'* divergence theorem as well as the *Cauchy stress lemma* the following is achieved:

$$\int_{\mathcal{B}_t} \left\{\rho\,(\mathbf{x}, t)\,\mathbf{a} - \mathrm{div}\boldsymbol{\sigma}^T - \mathbf{b}\,(\mathbf{x}, t)\right\}\;dv = 0. \tag{3.18}$$

  For a constant velocity field the acceleration is zero, $\mathbf{a} = 0$, and thus the equilibrium equation reduces to

$$\mathrm{div}\boldsymbol{\sigma}^T + \mathbf{b}\,(\mathbf{x}, t) = 0. \tag{3.19}$$

  Following the same steps, the equilibrium equation for constant motion in the undeformed configuration, known as the *Lagrangian equation of motion*, is given by

$$\mathrm{div}\boldsymbol{P} + \mathbf{b}\,(\mathbf{X}, t) = 0. \tag{3.20}$$

  The balance of angular momentum is defined as a moment of the linear momentum taken about a particular point, and this energy form must be conserved too.

- **Conservation of energy:** The principle law of energy conservation dictates that energy cannot be created nor destroyed - it merely changes form. Energy has numerous categories, such as kinetic, mechanical, electrical, thermal and gravitational energies. However, this project only considers the conversion of energy into deformations, known as elastic potential energy.

## 3.4 Variation formulation

The variational principles for classical continua are used to solve a coupled system of nonlinear partial differential equations involving deformation and strain measures. Cardiac mechanics problems can be analyzed using these variational principles, though such problems are geometrically complex and require computational solving techniques. This research uses the Element-Free Galerkin (EFG) method - a derivative of the Finite Element Method (FEM) - which is based on the variational principles of the governing equations, often referred to as the weak form or the principle of virtual work.

For classical continua considering deformations only, a single-field variational principle $\delta\Psi(\mathbf{u})$ for an unknown displacement field for classical degrees of freedom $\mathbf{u}$ is utilized. A material body $\mathcal{B}$ needs external energy transferred to it in order for it to deform and thus store that supplied energy internally by deforming. The external work $\mathcal{W}_{ext}$ acting on a body comprises of a body force $\mathbf{b}$ that can act over the volume of the body $\mathcal{B}$, and surface force $\mathbf{t}^{(\mathbf{n})}$ acting on the boundary $\partial\mathcal{B}_N$ of the body with unit surface normal vector $\mathbf{n}$. The external forces are catered for by a *boundary value problem*, which comprises of two distinct boundary condition types: the *Dirichlet boundary conditions* of prescribed deformations $\mathbf{u} = \bar{\mathbf{u}}$ occurring on $\partial\mathcal{B}_D \subset \partial\mathcal{B}$, such as support reactions, and the *Neumann boundary conditions* of prescribed tractions $\mathbf{t}^{(\mathbf{n})}$ occurring on $\partial\mathcal{B}_N$, such as surface pressures. These two boundary conditions share the following linkage:

$$\partial\mathcal{B} = \partial\mathcal{B}_N \cup \partial\mathcal{B}_D \quad \text{and} \quad \partial\mathcal{B}_N \cap \partial\mathcal{B}_D = \emptyset. \tag{3.21}$$

The strain energy function $\psi(\mathbf{E})$ is used to quantify the internal work generated as a function of the *Green* strain tensor $\mathbf{E}$ expressed as

$$\mathcal{W}_{int}(\mathbf{u}) = \int_{\mathcal{B}} \frac{\partial\psi(\mathbf{E})}{\partial\mathbf{E}} : \delta\mathbf{E}\, dV = \int_{\mathcal{B}} \mathbf{S} : \delta\mathbf{E}\, dV. \tag{3.22}$$

The external work done by body forces $\mathbf{b}$ on $\mathcal{B}$ and prescribed surface tractions $\mathbf{t}^{(\mathbf{n})}$ on $\partial\mathcal{B}_N$ is given by

$$\mathcal{W}_{ext}(\mathbf{u}) = \int_{\mathcal{B}} \rho_0\mathbf{b} \cdot \delta\mathbf{u}\, dV + \int_{\delta\mathcal{B}_N} \mathbf{t}^{(\mathbf{n})} \cdot \delta\mathbf{u}\, dA. \tag{3.23}$$

The conservation of energy is also maintained in the variational formulation, and as such the total external work expended on a body is equal to the total internal work stored in that body. The full variational formulation is therefore represented as

$$\delta\Psi(\mathbf{u}) = \mathcal{W}_{int} - \mathcal{W}_{ext} = 0 \tag{3.24}$$

$$= \int_{\mathcal{B}} \mathbf{S} : \delta\mathbf{E}\, dV - \int_{\mathcal{B}} \rho_0\mathbf{b} \cdot \delta\mathbf{u}\, dV - \int_{\delta\mathcal{B}_N} \mathbf{t}^{(\mathbf{n})} \cdot \delta\mathbf{u}\, dA = 0 \tag{3.25}$$

where $\mathbf{u} = \bar{\mathbf{u}}$ on $\partial\mathcal{B}_D$. For a more detailed description of the variational formulation the reader is referred to Wriggers [94], Holzapfel [34], and Fish [20].

## 3.5 Classical constitutive law

The kinematic relations, stresses and balance laws presented thus far remain valid for all branches of continuum mechanics; however, they do not distinguish between one material and another. A constitutive law representative of the material is required in order to achieve a full set of equations to solve a boundary value problem. The constitutive law serves to express the stress components developed in a body $\mathcal{B}$ in terms of other field functions, typically strain. The stress and strain relationship in materials can be extremely complex, particularly for biological materials, with nonlinear stress responses to applied strain. The stress and strain developed in a material can be established experimentally, and a constitutive equation is used to relate the measured stress to the measured strain.

The phenomenological approach involves the calibration of a constitutive law to reproduce experimental data, which can then be used to approximate the stress caused by all deformations of the material, with the quality of the approximation dependent on the intricacy of the material behaviour and the sophistication of the constitutive equation used to describe such behaviour. For instance, if the material behaves linearly then a simple linear constitutive function might adequately approximate the stresses developed in a material. However, in the case of cardiac modelling, a more complex constitutive law is required, as it was found that cardiac tissue behaves nonlinearly, and further responds differently depending on the direction along which the material was deformed [81, 12]. In order to comment on the suitability and versatility of a micromorphic material model for cardiac tissue modelling, its performance against existing classical models must be scrutinized.

There are three types of constitutive equations that can be used to model cardiac tissue: isotropy, transverse isotropy and orthotropy. If the material does not exhibit directional dependence from its stress response, then it is deemed isotropic. The material is transversely isotropic if it has one preferred material direction of differing properties from the bulk material, with the plane perpendicular to the preferred direction being isotropic. Finally, a material is orthotropic if it has unique responses along three preferred orthogonal material directions.

From data collected by Sommer et al. (2015) and Rohmer et al. (2007) for human cardiac tissue, as well as porcine [12], canine [52], rat [77], sheep [28] and bovine [24] studies, it is evident that cardiac tissue has complex architecture and deformation modes along all three of its unique material directions. Though transverse isotropy is often the first step in modelling anisotropic materials, it was omitted in place of more versatile orthotropy, as guided by the findings of Usyk et al. (2000). It was observed by both Sommer et al. (2015) and Dokos et al. (2002) that not only is cardiac tissue orthotropic, but it also produces non-linear deformations. Cardiac tissue requires lower proportional stresses for low strains, than it does for higher strains, and thus the stress grows exponentially for prescribed deformations. Furthermore, myocardial tissue is only slightly compressible, therefore a suitable constitutive law would need to cater for this near incompressibility [96].

There are three orthonormal material covariant directions of myocardial tissue: the muscle fibres $\mathbf{V}_f$, the sheets containing the muscle fibres $\mathbf{V}_s$ and its sheet-normal direction $\mathbf{V}_n$. Together they form the bases of a local *Green strain* tensor $\mathbf{E}$ set in the orthonormal basis $(\mathbf{V}_f, \mathbf{V}_s, \mathbf{V}_n)$ such that

$$\begin{aligned}\mathbf{E} = {} & E_{ff}\mathbf{V}^f \otimes \mathbf{V}^f + E_{ss}\mathbf{V}^s \otimes \mathbf{V}^s + E_{nn}\mathbf{V}^n \otimes \mathbf{V}^n + E_{fs}\left(\mathbf{V}^f \otimes \mathbf{V}^s + \mathbf{V}^s \otimes \mathbf{V}^f\right) \\ & + E_{fn}\left(\mathbf{V}^f \otimes \mathbf{V}^n + \mathbf{V}^n \otimes \mathbf{V}^f\right) + E_{sn}\left(\mathbf{V}^s \otimes \mathbf{V}^n + \mathbf{V}^n \otimes \mathbf{V}^s\right). \end{aligned} \tag{3.26}$$

This local *Green strain* tensor $\mathbf{E}$ was used by Usyk et al. (2000) to formulate the left ventricular passive filling constitutive law $\psi_{[\text{pass.}]}$, and was calibrated successfully for a canine left ventricle in [87, 88]. The formulation uses a *Fung*-type exponential constitutive equation developed in previous studies of [22, 4, 41, 40]. The following constitutive law encompasses both the orthotropy and non-linearity $_{[\text{orth./exp.}]}$, as well as the near incompressibility $\psi_{[\text{comp.}]}$ of the material, and was thus adopted for this study:

$$\psi_{[\text{pass.}]} = \psi_{[\text{orth./exp.}]} + \psi_{[\text{comp.}]} = \frac{1}{2}A\left(e^{Q} - 1\right) + A_{\text{comp}}\left[J\,ln(J) - J + 1\right], \tag{3.27}$$

where

$$Q = b_{ff}E_{ff}^2 + b_{ss}E_{ss}^2 + b_{nn}E_{nn}^2 + b_{fs}\left(E_{fs}^2 + E_{sf}^2\right) + b_{fn}\left(E_{fn}^2 + E_{nf}^2\right) + b_{sn}\left(E_{sn}^2 + E_{ns}^2\right). \tag{3.28}$$

In Eq. (3.28) the material parameters $b_{ij}$ determine the material anisotropy, and in Eq. (3.27) $J$ is the Jacobian, the parameter $A$ is used as a global stress scaling coefficient, and $A_{\text{comp}}$ is the compressibility coefficient.

Legner et al. (2014) adapted $Q$ to an invariant based approach [51], which uses structural tensors

$$\mathbf{M}_f = \mathbf{V}_f \otimes \mathbf{V}_f; \quad \mathbf{M}_s = \mathbf{V}_s \otimes \mathbf{V}_s; \quad \mathbf{M}_n = \mathbf{V}_n \otimes \mathbf{V}_n, \tag{3.29}$$

where

$$\begin{aligned} Q^{Inv.} &= a_1\left(\text{tr}(\mathbf{M}_f\mathbf{E})\right)^2 + a_2\left(\text{tr}(\mathbf{M}_s\mathbf{E})\right)^2 + a_3\left(\text{tr}(\mathbf{M}_n\mathbf{E})\right)^2 \\ &\quad + a_4\,\text{tr}\left(\mathbf{M}_f(\mathbf{E})^2\right) + a_5\,\text{tr}\left(\mathbf{M}_s(\mathbf{E})^2\right) + a_6\,\text{tr}\left(\mathbf{M}_n(\mathbf{E})^2\right). \end{aligned} \tag{3.30}$$

Legner et al. motivated that the invariant approach is easier to implement; however, the problem it creates is that the material parameters $a_i$ have overlapping contributions to different shear modes, and as such it is harder to grasp what each parameter represents physically. Further, it is more difficult to enforce convexity requirements discussed by Wilber and Walton (2002) using $a_i$, whereas it is straightforward to enforce with $b_{ij} > 0$. It is possible to relate material parameters $a_i$ in terms of $b_{ij}$ as follows

$$\begin{aligned} a_1 &= b_{ff} - b_{fs} - b_{fn} + b_{sn} & a_4 &= b_{fs} + b_{fn} - b_{sn} \\ a_2 &= b_{ss} - b_{fs} + b_{fn} - b_{sn} & a_5 &= b_{fs} - b_{fn} + b_{sn} \\ a_3 &= b_{nn} + b_{fs} - b_{fn} - b_{sn} & a_6 &= -b_{fs} + b_{fn} + b_{sn} \end{aligned} \tag{3.31}$$

Finally, the constitutive equation relating the passive stress $\mathbf{S}^{(Pass.)}$ response of cardiac tissue to strain is given as

$$\mathbf{S}^{(Pass.)} = \frac{\partial\psi}{\partial\mathbf{E}}. \tag{3.32}$$

It is also possible to use classical mechanics to model heterogeneous, or more particularly fibrous, materials using the rule of mixtures, such as the studies on urinary bladder tissue [61] and brain tissue [13]. For the rule of mixtures we find the stress contributions in the composite material ($E_c\epsilon_c$) can be separated additively into that of the fibres ($E_f\epsilon_f$) and that of the material matrix ($E_m\epsilon_m$):

$$E_c\epsilon_c = fE_f\epsilon_f + (1 - f)\,E_m\epsilon_m, \tag{3.33}$$

where $f$ is the volume fraction of the fibres compared with the total material volume. The use of the rule of mixtures provides the computational efficiency of classical mechanics, however, we find that the strain between the matrix and fibre is constrained such that $\epsilon_m = \epsilon_f$, and hence it would not be possible to get independent motion of the muscle fibres relative to the matrix using this process. Conversely, the micromorphic approach should allow for non-affine motion of the muscle fibres, and hence offers greater versatility to capture cardiac mechanics.

# 4

# Micromorphic Continuum Theory

A micromorphic continuum falls under the category of continuum theories and was conceived in the theoretical considerations of Ericksen and Truesdell (1957), but it was the seminal work of Eringen and Suhubi (1964) that devised its terminology and firmly established the theory in its sphere of research [78]. Micromorphic theory is part of an exciting field of multiscale continuum theories which attempt to incorporate the internal architecture of a material on a so-called micro-scale. In a micromorphic continuum, the average of all the micro-volumes $dV'$ produces a continuous mass distribution at each point of the macro-element $dV$, and hence gives the total mass $dM$ and adheres to continuum theory [15]. Eringen's definition of a micro-continuum is a continuous collection of deformable point particles, also referred to as fibres or micro-directors [18]. It is possible to attribute different properties to these particles, and in turn develop sophisticated material behaviour.

This research explores the novel interpretation of the micromorphic theory proposed by Sansour (1998), which attempts to overcome shortfalls in Eringen and Suhubi's strain measures in terms of Euler-Lagrange equations by supplementing new strain measures and corresponding field equations. This section outlines the fundamental concepts of the micromorphic model in terms of kinematics and stress, and then expands upon the interpretation of Sansour to include the subsequent work of Sansour and Skatulla (2009) and a quadratic approach in Sansour et al. (2010). Finally, the author's own interpretation of the micromorphic model is outlined to address potential numerical artifacts in Sansour's micromorphic model with respect to its micro-director displacements and handling of micro-boundary conditions observed in this study.

## 4.1 Kinematics of the micromorphic continuum

Micromorphic theory depicts a material body as a continuous compilation of deformable particles, with each particle having finite size and inner structure. The micromorphic continuum goes beyond the classical continuum of infinitesimal size and no inner structure, to take into consideration the microstructure of a material whilst maintaining the advantages of continuum theory. The classical deformable point is replaced by a micromorphic point, which is a geometric point containing an additional set of vectors used to describe the orientations and deformations of all the component materials that constitute the collective material [50], as depicted in Figure 4.1.

The following definitions, notation and terminology follow the conventions as per Eringen (1999), and serve to introduce the micromorphic model using Eringen's description. A material point $P(\mathbf{X}, \Xi)$ is described by its centroid $\mathbf{X}$ and vector (micro-director) $\boldsymbol{\Xi}$ bound to $\mathbf{X}$, as seen in Figure 4.1. The point $\mathbf{X}$ is described by rectangular coordinates $X_1, X_2, X_3$ in a coordinate frame $X_K, K = 1, 2, 3$, and the vector $\boldsymbol{\Xi}$ with components $\Xi_K(\Xi_1, \Xi_2, \Xi_3)$ in the same coordinate frame $X_K$ [18]. The material point $P(\mathbf{X}, \boldsymbol{\Xi})$ undergoes deformation to its spatial point $P(\mathbf{x}, \boldsymbol{\xi})$ such that

$$X_K \to x_k = x_k(X_k, t) \tag{4.1}$$

$$\Xi_K \to \xi_k = \xi_k(X_k, \Xi_k, t), \tag{4.2}$$

where the *macro-motion* of $x_k$ in Eq. (4.1) accounts for the motion of the centroid of the particle, and the *micro-motion* of $\xi_k$ in Eq. (4.2) accounts for the motion of the inner structure. Eringen's *definition 1* of a micromorphic continuum states that a material body is deemed a micromorphic continuum if its motion is described by Eq. (4.1) and Eq. (4.2) which maintain continuous partial derivatives with respect to $X_K$ and $t$, and which are invertible uniquely. It is possible to map the deformation of the inner structure of the particle using a micro-deformation tensor $\chi_{kK}$, and because the material particles are infinitesimally small compared to macroscopic scales of the body, a linear approximation in $\boldsymbol{\Xi}$ is permissible

$$\xi_k = \chi_{kK}(\mathbf{X}, t)\Xi_K. \tag{4.3}$$

In addition to the three classical displacement degrees of freedom of the centroid of a particle, the micromorphic material also has nine independent degrees of freedom for both stretches and rotations defined in the micro-deformation tensor $\chi_{kK}$. The axiom of continuity, which stipulates that matter is indestructible and impenetrable, is upheld by the macro-motion Jacobian $J$ and the micro-motion Jacobian $j$ both enforced as strictly positive [91].

$$J \equiv \det(x_{k,K}) > 0 \qquad \text{and} \qquad j \equiv \det(\chi_{kK}) > 0 \tag{4.4}$$

Eringen set out the polynomial that can be used to describe the *intrinsic motion* (micro-motion), $\boldsymbol{\xi}$, in terms of $\boldsymbol{\Xi}$:

$$\boldsymbol{\xi} = \boldsymbol{\chi}_K(\mathbf{X}, t)\,\boldsymbol{\Xi}_K + \frac{1}{2}\boldsymbol{\chi}_{KL}(\mathbf{X}, t)\,\boldsymbol{\Xi}_K\boldsymbol{\Xi}_L + \dots. \tag{4.5}$$

However, Eringen did stress that the use of just the first micro-deformation gradient $\boldsymbol{\chi}_K$ or $\chi_{kK}$ is already complicated, and thus the use of higher-order micro-deformation gradients is questionable and impractical [16].

We now progress to the micromorphic theory of Sansour (1998), which will form the basis of the model developed in this study, and thus all subsequent micromorphic notation in this study will follow Sansour's conventions. Sansour proposed that a generalized micromorphic continuum $\mathcal{G}$ is constructed by the Cartesian product of a macro-space $\mathcal{B} \in \mathbb{E}(3)$ (parameterized by curvilinear coordinates $\vartheta^p$) and a micro-space $\mathcal{S}$ (parameterized by curvilinear coordinates $\zeta^\beta$). Henceforth, the Latin indices represent the macro-dimensions, and the Greek indices represent the micro-dimensions. In the case of a three-dimensional macro-space we write the generalized micromorphic continuum as

$$\mathcal{G} := \mathcal{B} \times \mathcal{S} \subset \mathbb{E}(3 + n), \tag{4.6}$$

where the micro-space is $n$-dimensional to match the topology of the micro-structure. This is highly advantageous as an infinite number of additional degrees of freedom can be added to every point of the basic continuum [73]. Furthermore, this generalized continuum definition allows us to integrate over the macro and micro continua separately [74]. The micro-dimensions only refer to each vector adding detail to the micro-structure, and these vectors are henceforth referred to interchangeably as micro-dimensions, micro-directors or micro-coordinates. It must be clarified that although the micro-space is referred to as $n$-dimensional or as having $n$ micro-directors, we find the number of degrees of freedom for each micro-director must still match the number of degrees of freedom of the macro-space, in order for the micro-director to be orientated in the continuum. For example, in a two-dimensional macro-space with a one-dimensional micro-space, we find a single micro-director that has two degrees of freedom relative to $X_1, X_2$ to orientate the micro-director in the continuum. Similarly, in a three-dimensional macro-space with in a five-dimensional micro-space, we find the five micro-directors will each have three degrees of freedom relative to $X_1, X_2, X_3$ to orientate the micro-directors in the continuum.

### 4.1.1 Deformation measures

The deformation measures used to describe Sansour's generalized micromorphic continuum are outlined in this section. We assume that the micromorphic placement vector $\tilde{\mathbf{X}}$ of a material point $P(\tilde{\mathbf{X}} \in \mathcal{G})$ is of an additive nature and is the aggregate of its location in the macro-continuum $\mathbf{X} \in \mathcal{B}$ and in the micro-continuum $\mathbf{\Xi} \in \mathcal{S}$. The macro-placement vector $\mathbf{X}$ describes the origin of the micro-coordinate system, in order for the micro-director $\mathbf{\Xi}$ to be relative to the macro-placement. The macro-placement $\mathbf{X}$ is defined as a function of the macro-coordinates $\vartheta^p$ only, whereas $\mathbf{\Xi}$ is defined a function of both the macro-coordinates $\vartheta^p$ and the micro-coordinates $\zeta^\beta$ [75].

$$\tilde{\mathbf{X}} = \mathbf{X}(\vartheta^p) + \mathbf{\Xi}(\vartheta^p, \zeta^\beta) \quad \text{(Reference configuration)} \tag{4.7}$$

Similarly, in the deformed configuration we assume that the micromorphic placement vector $\tilde{\mathbf{x}}$ of a spatial point $p(\tilde{\mathbf{x}} \in \mathcal{G}_t)$ is the sum of its position in the macro-continuum $\mathbf{x} \in \mathcal{B}_t$ and in the micro-continuum $\boldsymbol{\xi} \in \mathcal{S}_t$.

$$\tilde{\mathbf{x}} = \mathbf{x}(\vartheta^p, t) + \boldsymbol{\xi}(\vartheta^p, \zeta^\beta, t) \quad \text{(Deformed configuration)} \tag{4.8}$$

The unique one-to-one mapping of a micromorphic material point $\tilde{\mathbf{X}}$ to the corresponding spatial point $\tilde{\mathbf{x}}$, as seen in Figure(4.1), is achieved in accordance with the impenetrability and indestructibility of matter by $\tilde{\varphi} : \mathcal{G} \to \mathcal{G}_t$ to give

$$\tilde{\mathbf{x}} = \tilde{\varphi}\left(\tilde{\mathbf{X}}, t\right), \quad \text{and} \quad \tilde{\mathbf{X}} = \tilde{\varphi}^{-1}(\tilde{\mathbf{x}}, t). \tag{4.9}$$

#### 4.1.1.1 Linear approach

The most basic micromorphic particle is that of a linear ansatz, also suggested by Eringen [18]. The micro-director is orientated through the material vector function of unit length $\mathbf{a}^0_\alpha(\vartheta^p, \zeta^\beta)$ or its spatial equivalent $\mathbf{a}_\alpha(\vartheta^p, \zeta^\beta, t)$, providing together with the micro-coordinate $\zeta^\alpha$ the micro-space placement in reference and current configuration, respectively

$$\mathbf{\Xi} = \zeta^\alpha \mathbf{a}^0_\alpha(\vartheta^p, \zeta^\beta), \quad \text{and} \quad \boldsymbol{\xi} = \zeta^\alpha \mathbf{a}_\alpha(\vartheta^p, \zeta^\beta, t), \tag{4.10}$$

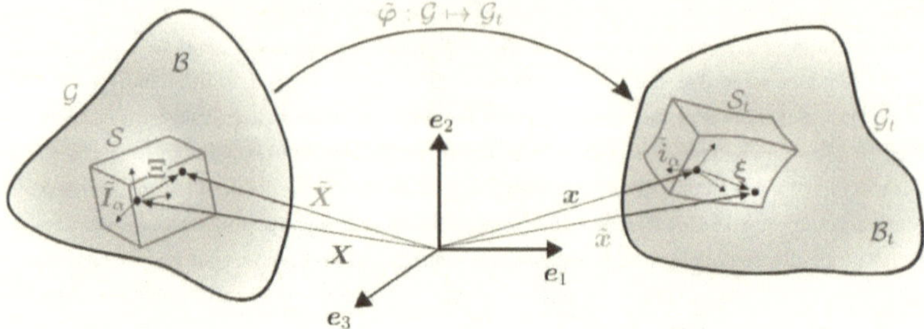


Fig. 4.1: Macro-motions and micro-motions of a micromorphic particle from the reference configuration to the deformed configuration [90].

where the index $\alpha = 1, n$ for an $n$-dimensional micro-space, or $n$ micro-directors. The micromorphic placement in the combined macro-space and micro-space is then defined according to Eq. (4.7) and Eq. (4.8) in either configuration as

$$\tilde{\mathbf{X}} = \mathbf{X}(\vartheta^p) + \zeta^\alpha \mathbf{a}^0_\alpha(\vartheta^p, \zeta^\beta) \tag{4.11}$$

$$\tilde{\mathbf{x}} = \mathbf{x}(\vartheta^p, t) + \zeta^\alpha \mathbf{a}_\alpha(\vartheta^p, \zeta^\beta, t). \tag{4.12}$$

As with the classical displacement field $\mathbf{u}(\mathbf{X}, t)$, we introduce a micro-deformation $\mathbf{w}_\alpha(\vartheta^p, \zeta^\beta, t)$ such that

$$\mathbf{w}_\alpha(\vartheta^p, \zeta^\beta, t) = \mathbf{a}_\alpha(\vartheta^p, \zeta^\beta, t) - \mathbf{a}^0_\alpha(\vartheta^p, \zeta^\beta). \tag{4.13}$$

In the most general form the micro-directors are not uniform through $\mathcal{B}$ and $\mathcal{S}$, as is the case with most biological materials. For the purpose of micromorphic cardiac tissue mechanics, we can identify each $\mathbf{a}^0_\alpha$ at time $t = 0$ with the orientation of the myocardial muscle fibre/fibre bundle $\mathbf{V}^f$ in the undeformed/unloaded configuration at the generalized placement $\tilde{\mathbf{X}}$. The dependency of $\mathbf{a}_\alpha$ on the micro-coordinate $\zeta^\alpha$ stems from the fact that the orientation of the micro-space is capable of varying in $\mathcal{S}$. This fact is crucial when the influence of the spatially changing anisotropy of the tissue needs to be addressed on the micro-scale. The principle merits of the micromorphic model to replicate characteristic features of cardiac tissue can be adequately explored using this linear model. In fact, the inherent complexities of the micromorphic model make it preferable to use a simplified version of the model at this stage of analysis, as additional terms make understanding the contributions of the micromorphic model harder to isolate and decipher.

#### 4.1.1.2 Quadratic approach

The linear ansatz of Eq. (4.11) and Eq. (4.12) produce a second strain measure that is not full rank [75]. To achieve full rank the approach is extended to a quadratic formulation as per Sansour et al. (2010), where a further set of micro-vectors $\mathbf{b}_{\alpha\beta}$ provides extra degrees of freedom.

$$\tilde{\mathbf{x}} = \mathbf{x}\left(\vartheta^p, t\right) + \zeta^\alpha \mathbf{a}_\alpha\left(\vartheta^p, \zeta^\beta, t\right) + \zeta^\alpha\, \zeta^\beta \mathbf{b}_{\alpha\beta}\left(\vartheta^p, t\right) \tag{4.14}$$

This formulation requires many extra degrees of freedom; however, it is possible to simplify the micromorphic placement vector with fewer degrees of freedom as follows

$$\tilde{\mathbf{x}} = \mathbf{x}\left(\vartheta^p, t\right) + \zeta^\alpha \, \left(1 + \zeta^\beta \, \chi_\beta\left(\vartheta^p, t\right)\right) \, \mathbf{a}_\alpha\left(\vartheta^p, \zeta^\beta, t\right) \, . \tag{4.15}$$

The scalar field $\chi_\alpha\left(\vartheta^p, t\right)$ provides one extra non-physical degree of freedom per micro-director [89], and is introduced to achieve strain measures of full rank with $\chi_\beta^{(t=0)} = 0$. Eq. (4.14) is simplified to give only 4 extra degrees of freedom for each micro-director in Eq. (4.15), and the extra degrees of freedom are constant in $\mathcal{S}$. The quadratic approach was successfully implemented by the author, but it was not investigated in this study due to anticipated complexity in attributing material response to its more numerous strain measures compared with the less complicated linear approach. However, the quadratic approach was employed in the numerical examples of von Hoegen et al. (2017), which will be used for comparison and validation of certain results from the linear approach used in this research.

#### 4.1.1.3 Spatial derivatives

In order to formulate the strain measures used to describe the kinematics, the spatial derivatives of the macro-placement and micro-placement vectors are required. The derivative of the linear ansatz of $\tilde{\mathbf{x}}$ in Eq. (4.12) with respect to the macro coordinates $\vartheta^p$ is

$$\tilde{\mathbf{x}}_{,p} = \frac{\partial \tilde{\mathbf{x}}}{\partial \vartheta^p} = \mathbf{x}_{,p} + \zeta^\alpha \mathbf{a}_{\alpha,p} \, , \tag{4.16}$$

and the derivative with respect to the micro-coordinates $\zeta^\alpha$ is

$$\tilde{\mathbf{x}}_{,\gamma} = \frac{\partial \tilde{\mathbf{x}}}{\partial \zeta^\gamma} = \frac{\partial \zeta^\alpha}{\partial \zeta^\gamma} \mathbf{a}_\alpha = \delta^{\alpha}_{\cdot\gamma} \mathbf{a}_\alpha = \mathbf{a}_\gamma . \tag{4.17}$$

In the generic formulation up to this point, $\mathbf{a}_\alpha$ was also a function of the micro-space, and therefore could have its own micro-derivative $\mathbf{a}_{\alpha,\gamma}$. However, this was omitted in this study and it was considered that higher-order contributions were not essential to assess the capabilities of the micromorphic model.

#### 4.1.1.4 Tangent space

The tangent space $\mathcal{TG}$ in the reference configuration stems from the covariant curvilinear (natural) basis vectors of the macro-scale $\mathcal{TB}$ and micro-scale $\mathcal{TS}$ pair $(\tilde{\mathbf{G}}_p \times \tilde{\mathbf{I}}_\alpha)$ given by

$$\tilde{\mathbf{G}}_p = \frac{\partial \tilde{\mathbf{X}}}{\partial \vartheta^p} \quad (p = \text{macro-coordinates}); \quad \text{and} \quad \tilde{\mathbf{I}}_\alpha = \frac{\partial \tilde{\mathbf{X}}}{\partial \zeta^\alpha} \quad (\alpha = \text{micro-coordinates}). \tag{4.18}$$

The corresponding dual contravariant natural basis vectors are expressed as $\tilde{\mathbf{G}}^p$ and $\tilde{\mathbf{I}}^\alpha$, and can be calculated using the following property

$$\tilde{\mathbf{G}}_p \cdot \tilde{\mathbf{G}}^q = \delta_{p}^{\cdot q}, \qquad \tilde{\mathbf{I}}_\alpha \cdot \tilde{\mathbf{I}}^\beta = \delta_{\alpha}^{\cdot\beta}. \tag{4.19}$$

The associated tangent space $\mathcal{TG}_t$ in the deformed configuration is spanned by the curvilinear basis vectors of the macro-scale $\mathcal{TB}_t$ and micro-scale $\mathcal{TS}_t$ pair $(\tilde{\mathbf{g}}_p \times \tilde{\mathbf{i}}_\alpha)$ given by

$$\tilde{\mathbf{g}}_p = \frac{\partial \tilde{\mathbf{x}}}{\partial \vartheta^p} \quad \text{and} \quad \tilde{\mathbf{i}}_\alpha = \frac{\partial \tilde{\mathbf{x}}}{\partial \zeta^\alpha}. \tag{4.20}$$

It is important to establish that the tangent space is not trivial. The tangent of the projection maps depends on the topology of the micro-space, and thus could allow for a curvature or complicated microstructure to give a non-trivial projection map. Further, the tangent of the projection map defines the conversion metrics used to evaluate the integrals over the micro-space found in the variational formulation. In order to compensate for such complexities, the tangent space is elaborated as follows

$$\tilde{\mathbf{G}}_p = \frac{\partial \tilde{\mathbf{X}}}{\partial \vartheta^p} = \frac{\partial (\mathbf{X} + \zeta^\beta \mathbf{a}^0_\beta)}{\partial \vartheta^p} = \mathbf{V}_p + \zeta^\beta \, \mathbf{a}^0_{\beta,p}. \tag{4.21}$$

In this study the standard case of a Cartesian coordinate system for the macro-space was used, and therefore $\vartheta^p = X_k$. Furthermore, the higher-order contributions of $\zeta^\beta \, \mathbf{a}^{(0)}_{\beta,p}$ were deemed higher-order and ignored from the basis vector, resulting in the trivial case

$$\tilde{\mathbf{G}}_p = \mathbf{e}_p. \tag{4.22}$$

For the micro-scale we elaborate on the tangent space as follows

$$\tilde{\mathbf{I}}_\alpha = \frac{\partial \tilde{\mathbf{X}}}{\partial \zeta^\alpha} = \frac{\partial (\mathbf{X} + \zeta^\beta \mathbf{a}^0_\beta)}{\partial \zeta^\alpha} = \frac{\partial (\zeta^\beta \mathbf{a}^0_\beta)}{\partial \zeta^\alpha} = \delta^\beta_{.\alpha} \mathbf{a}^0_\beta = \mathbf{a}^0_\alpha. \tag{4.23}$$

#### 4.1.1.5 Generalized deformation gradient

To extract the various micromorphic strain measures to come, it is necessary to first describe the *generalized deformation gradient* $\tilde{\mathbf{F}}$ as

$$\begin{aligned}
\tilde{\mathbf{F}} &= \frac{\partial \tilde{\mathbf{x}}}{\partial \tilde{\mathbf{X}}} = \frac{\partial \mathbf{x}}{\partial \tilde{\mathbf{X}}} + \frac{\partial \boldsymbol{\xi}}{\partial \tilde{\mathbf{X}}} \\
&= \frac{\partial \mathbf{x}}{\partial \vartheta^k} \otimes \frac{\partial \vartheta^k}{\partial \tilde{\mathbf{X}}} + \frac{\partial \boldsymbol{\xi}}{\partial \zeta^\alpha} \otimes \frac{\partial \zeta^\alpha}{\partial \tilde{\mathbf{X}}} \\
&= \frac{\partial \mathbf{x}}{\partial \vartheta^k} \otimes \tilde{\mathbf{G}}^k + \frac{\partial \boldsymbol{\xi}}{\partial \zeta^\alpha} \otimes \tilde{\mathbf{I}}^\alpha .
\end{aligned} \tag{4.24}$$

We then substitute in the macro and micro spatial derivative of Eq. (4.16) and Eq. (4.17), respectively

$$\tilde{\mathbf{F}} = (\mathbf{x}_{,i} + \zeta^\alpha \mathbf{a}_{\alpha,i}) \otimes \tilde{\mathbf{G}}^i + \mathbf{a}_\gamma \otimes \tilde{\mathbf{I}}^\gamma . \tag{4.25}$$

### 4.1.2 Strain measures

In accordance with the definition of the classical right *Cauchy-Green* deformation tensor, the generalized right *Cauchy-Green* deformation tensor $\tilde{\mathbf{C}}$ is calculated using the generalized deformation gradient of Eq. (4.25) as follows

$$\tilde{\mathbf{C}} = \tilde{\mathbf{F}}^T \tilde{\mathbf{F}}, \tag{4.26}$$

and ignoring higher-order (quadratic) terms of $\zeta^\alpha$ we find

$$\begin{aligned}
\tilde{\mathbf{C}} &= \left[\mathbf{x}_{,i}\mathbf{x}_{,j} + \zeta^\alpha \mathbf{a}_{\alpha,i}\mathbf{x}_{,j} + \zeta^\alpha \mathbf{a}_{\alpha,j}\mathbf{x}_{,i}\right] \tilde{\mathbf{G}}^i \otimes \tilde{\mathbf{G}}^j \\
&+ \left[\mathbf{x}_{,j}\mathbf{a}_\gamma + \zeta^\alpha \mathbf{a}_{\alpha,j}\mathbf{a}_\gamma\right] \left(\tilde{\mathbf{G}}^j \otimes \tilde{\mathbf{I}}^\gamma + \tilde{\mathbf{I}}^\gamma \otimes \tilde{\mathbf{G}}^j\right) \\
&+ \left[\mathbf{a}_\gamma \mathbf{a}_\phi\right] \tilde{\mathbf{I}}^\gamma \otimes \tilde{\mathbf{I}}^\phi .
\end{aligned} \tag{4.27}$$

It is possible to decompose $\tilde{\mathbf{C}}$ into a lower-order part $\mathbf{C}$ without dependence on $\zeta^\alpha$, as well as a higher-order part $\mathbf{K}_\alpha$ dependent on $\zeta^\alpha$.

$$\tilde{\mathbf{C}} = \mathbf{C} + \zeta^\alpha \mathbf{K}_\alpha \tag{4.28}$$

Furthermore, the generalized strain can be separated into three types based on their natural basis vectors: the macro-scale strain $\tilde{\mathbf{C}}^{(0)}$ linked to $\mathcal{TB}$ ($\tilde{\mathbf{G}}^k \otimes \tilde{\mathbf{G}}^l$); the relation between the macro-scale and micro-scale - termed the mixed-scale strain $\tilde{\mathbf{C}}^{(1)}$ relating $\mathcal{TB} \leftrightarrow \mathcal{TS}$ ($\tilde{\mathbf{G}}^j \otimes \tilde{\mathbf{I}}^\gamma + \tilde{\mathbf{I}}^\gamma \otimes \tilde{\mathbf{G}}^j$); and the micro-scale strain $\tilde{\mathbf{C}}^{(2)}$ linked to $\mathcal{TS}$ ($\tilde{\mathbf{I}}^\gamma \otimes \tilde{\mathbf{I}}^\phi$) [74, 75]. These may also be referred to as macro-bases, mixed-bases and micro-bases, respectively. This distinction is most beneficial when formulating the constitutive law for modelling cardiac mechanics, because different constitutive equations can be applied to each scale, thus enriching the model. The strain measures of the three scales are

$$\tilde{\mathbf{C}}^{(0)} = \mathbf{C}^{(0)} + \zeta^\alpha \mathbf{K}_\alpha^{(0)}; \qquad \tilde{\mathbf{C}}^{(1)} = \mathbf{C}^{(1)} + \zeta^\alpha \mathbf{K}_\alpha^{(1)}; \qquad \tilde{\mathbf{C}}^{(2)} = \mathbf{C}^{(2)} + \zeta^\alpha \mathbf{K}_\alpha^{(2)}, \tag{4.29}$$

where the lower-order strain measures are

$$C_{kl}^{(0)} = (x_{r,k}\, x_{r,l})\; \tilde{\mathbf{G}}^k \otimes \tilde{\mathbf{G}}^l \tag{4.30}$$

$$C_{j\gamma}^{(1)} = (x_{r,j}\, a_{\gamma r})\; \left(\tilde{\mathbf{G}}^j \otimes \tilde{\mathbf{I}}^\gamma + \tilde{\mathbf{I}}^\gamma \otimes \tilde{\mathbf{G}}^j\right) \tag{4.31}$$

$$C_{\gamma\phi}^{(2)} = (a_{\gamma r}\, a_{\phi r})\; \tilde{\mathbf{I}}^\gamma \otimes \tilde{\mathbf{I}}^\phi, \tag{4.32}$$

and the higher-order strain measures are

$$K_{\alpha kl}^{(0)} = (a_{\alpha r,k}\, x_{r,l} + a_{\alpha r,l}\, x_{r,k})\; \tilde{\mathbf{G}}^k \otimes \tilde{\mathbf{G}}^l \tag{4.33}$$

$$K_{\alpha j\gamma}^{(1)} = (a_{\alpha r,j}\, a_{\gamma r})\; \left(\tilde{\mathbf{G}}^j \otimes \tilde{\mathbf{I}}^\gamma + \tilde{\mathbf{I}}^\gamma \otimes \tilde{\mathbf{G}}^j\right). \tag{4.34}$$

For the linear ansatz used in this study, the higher-order term on the micro-scale $\mathbf{K}_\alpha^{(2)}$ falls away. It is evident that the lower-order strain $\mathbf{C}^{(0)}$ is akin to the classical right *Cauchy-Green* deformation tensor, the mixed-scale lower-order strain $\mathbf{C}^{(1)}$ characterizes the stretch and shear between the macro and micro tangent spaces, and the micro-scale lower-order strain $\mathbf{C}^{(2)}$ describes the micro-director strain. The higher-order strains $\mathbf{K}_\alpha^{(0)}$ and $\mathbf{K}_\alpha^{(1)}$ account for scale dependent non-local fluctuations of the material response [90]. Generally, the loading applied to the heart causes deformation of its bulk material activating both the displacement field $\mathbf{u}$ and the micro-deformation $\mathbf{w}_\alpha$. The evolution of the displacements needs to be independently controlled by formulating a suitable constitutive law for the different parts of $\tilde{\mathbf{C}}$. We can thus formulate a micromorphic strain energy function as a function of the generalized *Green* strain tensor

$$\tilde{\psi} := \tilde{\psi}\left(\tilde{\mathbf{E}}^{(0)}, \tilde{\mathbf{E}}^{(1)}, \tilde{\mathbf{E}}^{(2)}\right) \tag{4.35}$$

where the generalized *Green* strain tensor is defined as

$$\tilde{\mathbf{E}}^{(i)} = \frac{1}{2}\left(\tilde{\mathbf{C}}^{(i)} - \tilde{\mathbf{C}}^{(i)0}\right). \tag{4.36}$$

## 4.2 Kinematics of the MDO micromorphic model

There were potential issues encountered during this study relating to the micro-director displacements when using Sansour's version of the micromorphic model. Subsequently, the author developed a different approach to alleviate these issues. The cause of these issues, and why it is believed the author's alternative approach could remedy such issues, will be discussed later in Section 5. However, for the sake of continuity the kinematics are set out here. The author maintains Sansour's extraction of $\zeta^\alpha$ from $\Xi$ in Eq. (4.10), but to simplify the model we treat $\zeta^\alpha$ directly as the material's internal length scale rather than a micro-coordinate in this study. Therefore, we describe the alternative micromorphic placement vector $\breve{\mathbf{x}}$, differentiated in notation with a breve, as follows

$$\breve{\mathbf{x}} = \mathbf{x}(\vartheta^p, t) + \zeta^\alpha \mathbf{a}_\alpha(\vartheta^p, t). \tag{4.37}$$

Unlike Sansour's interpretation of separate macro-derivatives and micro-derivatives, the author is of the opinion that it is more appropriate to use only the macro-derivative. The micro-directors are situated at macroscopic points $X$, and therefore the micro-directors change from one macroscopic point to the next; hence it is the belief of the author that only a macroscopic derivative is appropriate for calculating quadratic length strain measures $(\mathbf{C}, \mathbf{E})$ for the overall material. This also ties in with Eringen (1999)'s micromorphic continuum *definition 1* mentioned already in Section 4.1 that states the macro-motion and micro-motion both possess continuous partial derivatives with respect to $X_K$ and $t$, whereby $X_K$ implies macro-derivatives. One notices in Eq. (4.37) that $\mathbf{a}_\alpha(\vartheta^p, t)$ is no longer a function of $\zeta^\alpha$ as it was in Eq. (4.12), as the micro-derivative is dismissed from this interpretation. Now, the only desired spatial derivative is with respect to the macro coordinates $\vartheta^p$

$$\breve{\mathbf{x}}_{,p} = \frac{\partial \breve{\mathbf{x}}}{\partial \vartheta^p} = \mathbf{x}_{,p} + \zeta^\alpha \mathbf{a}_{\alpha,p}\,. \tag{4.38}$$

From here a so-called *macro-derivative only* (MDO) micromorphic model is developed by the author, whereby its parameters are notated with a breve. The MDO generalized deformation gradient $\breve{\mathbf{F}}$ is calculated as

$$\breve{\mathbf{F}} = (\mathbf{x}_{,i} + \zeta^\alpha \mathbf{a}_{\alpha,i}) \otimes \breve{\mathbf{G}}^i, \tag{4.39}$$

where, as done in Eq. (4.22), we take the trivial case for the basis vector

$$\breve{\mathbf{G}}_p = \frac{\partial \breve{\mathbf{X}}}{\partial \vartheta^p} \approx \mathbf{e}_p. \tag{4.40}$$

The MDO generalized right *Cauchy-Green* deformation tensor $\breve{\mathbf{C}} = \breve{\mathbf{F}}^T \breve{\mathbf{F}}$ to give

$$\begin{aligned} \breve{\mathbf{C}} &= \breve{\mathbf{x}}_{,m} \cdot \breve{\mathbf{x}}_{,n} = \breve{x}_{r,m} \breve{x}_{r,n} \breve{\mathbf{G}}^m \otimes \breve{\mathbf{G}}^n \\ &= \left(x_{r,m} + \zeta^\alpha a_{\alpha r,m}\right)\left(x_{r,n} + \zeta^\beta a_{\beta r,n}\right) \breve{\mathbf{G}}^m \otimes \breve{\mathbf{G}}^n \\ &= \left[x_{r,m} x_{r,n} + x_{r,n} \zeta^\alpha a_{\alpha r,m} + x_{r,m} \zeta^\beta a_{\beta r,n} + \zeta^\alpha \zeta^\beta a_{\alpha r,m} a_{\beta r,n}\right] \breve{\mathbf{G}}^m \otimes \breve{\mathbf{G}}^n \end{aligned} \tag{4.41}$$

We find in Eq. (4.41) that all the strain terms are collected into a single strain tensor $\breve{\mathbf{C}}$. However, there is then no flexibility in distinguishing the contributions of the different components of the fibrous material. It is more desirable to isolate the strain into three different scales; macro-scale $\breve{\mathbf{C}}^{(0)}$, mixed-scale $\breve{\mathbf{C}}^{(1)}$ and micro-scale $\breve{\mathbf{C}}^{(2)}$, as per the scale definitions in Section 4.1, in order to differentiate the constitutive law contributions of each scale. The bases vectors were used by Sansour and Skatulla (2009) and von Hoegen et al. (2016) to separate the scales, with von Hoegen et al. then attributing bulk material interaction with $(\tilde{\mathbf{G}} \otimes \tilde{\mathbf{G}})$, relative deformation between bulk material and fibres with $(\tilde{\mathbf{G}} \otimes \tilde{\mathbf{I}} + \tilde{\mathbf{I}} \otimes \tilde{\mathbf{G}})$, and the deformation of the fibres themselves with $(\tilde{\mathbf{I}} \otimes \tilde{\mathbf{I}})$. However, the author believes that this does not result in the correct demarcations of higher-order strains $\mathbf{K}_\alpha^{(i)}$ according to their description of what each scale should represent.

The author agrees that the classification of what the scales should represent physically is most logical and useful: the macro-scale strain representing bulk material against bulk material interaction; the mixed-scale representing bulk material against fibre interaction; and the micro-scale strain representing fibre deformations. However, if we accept this definition, the author proposes that the strain components of the generalized right *Cauchy-Green* deformation tensor can only be distinguished by its combination of macro-scale deformation measures $\mathbf{u}_i$ and/or micro-scale deformation measures $\mathbf{a}_\gamma/\mathbf{a}_{\gamma,i}$. To elaborate, a strain measure containing $\mathbf{u}_{,i} \cdot \mathbf{u}_{,j}$ has macro-scale deformation measures only and is thus a macro-scale strain measure, a strain measure containing $\mathbf{u}_{,i} \cdot \mathbf{a}_{\gamma,j}$ has both a macro-scale deformation measure and a micro-scale deformation measure and is thus a mixed-scale strain measure, and finally a strain measure containing $\mathbf{a}_{\gamma,i} \cdot \mathbf{a}_{\beta,j}$ has micro-scale deformation measures only and is thus a micro-scale strain measure.

For example, this opinion is contradictory to Sansour and Skatulla (2009) in Eq. (19) and von Hoegen et al. (2016) in Eq. (8) whereby the strain measure containing $\mathbf{u}_{,i} \cdot \mathbf{a}_{\gamma,j}$ was attributed to the macro-scale strain tensor $\mathbf{K}_\alpha^{(0)}$, despite containing both macro-scale and micro-scale deformation measures. Furthermore, the stiffness of a material is a result of the interaction of its constituents. In terms of a numerical model, the numerical stiffness is derived from the derivatives of the strain and stress measures, and dictates how the macro/micro degrees of freedom of one node affect the macro/micro degrees of freedom of a neighbouring node, and hence the relevant strain scale. This further supports the author's demarcation of strain scales. Also, it can be shown that $\mathbf{K}_\alpha^{(0)}$ does not interact with the macro-scale degrees of freedom only between nodes in the numerical stiffness, but should rather be a mixed-scale interaction.

We therefore define three separate strain measures from Eq. (4.41) of the MDO micromorphic model as follows

$$\breve{\mathbf{C}}^{(0)} = x_{r,m} x_{r,n} \breve{\mathbf{G}}^m \otimes \breve{\mathbf{G}}^n \tag{4.42}$$

$$\breve{\mathbf{C}}^{(1)} = \left( x_{r,n} \zeta^\alpha a_{\alpha r,m} + x_{r,m} \zeta^\beta a_{\beta r,n} \right) \breve{\mathbf{G}}^m \otimes \breve{\mathbf{G}}^n \tag{4.43}$$

$$\breve{\mathbf{C}}^{(2)} = \zeta^\alpha \zeta^\beta a_{\alpha r,m} a_{\beta r,n} \breve{\mathbf{G}}^m \otimes \breve{\mathbf{G}}^n. \tag{4.44}$$

The influence on the material deformation behaviour from $\breve{\mathbf{C}}^{(1)}$ and $\breve{\mathbf{C}}^{(2)}$ can be scaled by the chosen size of $\zeta^\alpha$, in order to make the fibre (micro-director) contribution as significant as desired to approximate the fibrous material. Again, we formulate the MDO micromorphic strain energy function as a function of the generalized *Green* strain tensor

$$\breve{\psi} := \breve{\psi}\left( \breve{\mathbf{E}}^{(0)}, \breve{\mathbf{E}}^{(1)}, \breve{\mathbf{E}}^{(2)} \right), \tag{4.45}$$

where the generalized *Green* strain tensor is defined as

$$\breve{\mathbf{E}}^{(i)} = \frac{1}{2}\left( \breve{\mathbf{C}}^{(i)} - \breve{\mathbf{C}}^{(i)0} \right). \tag{4.46}$$

## 4.3 Micromorphic variational formulation

This section builds upon the classical variational formulation discussed in Section 3.4, and applies the process to the micromorphic strain measures of the generalized right *Cauchy-Green* deformation tensor $\tilde{\mathbf{C}}$ from Section 4.1.2, and then also to the MDO generalized right *Cauchy-Green* deformation tensor $\breve{\mathbf{C}}$ from Section 4.2.

### 4.3.1 Generalized micromorphic variational formulation

Consider a non-linear boundary value problem in the domain $\mathcal{B} \times \mathcal{S}$, where a volume element $dV$ is of the macroscopic domain $\mathcal{B}$, with a surface element $dA$ on its corresponding boundary $\partial\mathcal{B}$, and accordingly, a micro-volume element $dS$ is of the microscopic domain $\mathcal{S}$ with its boundary confined by $\partial\mathcal{S}$. It is presupposed that the body under consideration $\mathcal{B} \times \mathcal{S}$ is hyperelastic and possesses an elastic potential $\tilde{\Psi}$ represented by the stored strain energy per unit volume $\tilde{\psi}(\tilde{\mathbf{C}}^{(0)}, \tilde{\mathbf{C}}^{(1)}, \tilde{\mathbf{C}}^{(2)})$ applied to the micro-space $\mathcal{S}$. The stored strain energy is additively decomposed $\tilde{\psi} = \tilde{\psi}^{(0)} + \tilde{\psi}^{(1)} + \tilde{\psi}^{(2)}$, and hence the generalized second *Piola-Kirchhoff* stress tensors:

$$\tilde{\mathbf{S}}^{(0)} = 2\,\frac{\partial\tilde{\psi}^{(0)}}{\partial\tilde{\mathbf{C}}^{(0)}}; \qquad \tilde{\mathbf{S}}^{(1)} = 2\,\frac{\partial\tilde{\psi}^{(1)}}{\partial\tilde{\mathbf{C}}^{(1)}}; \qquad \tilde{\mathbf{S}}^{(2)} = 2\,\frac{\partial\tilde{\psi}^{(2)}}{\partial\tilde{\mathbf{C}}^{(2)}}, \tag{4.47}$$

which confirms the necessary linkage between energy-conjugate stress and strain measures. The external forces acting on the body are the body macro-forces $\mathbf{b}$ and body micro-forces $\mathbf{l}_\alpha$, as well as the boundary macro-tractions $\hat{\mathbf{t}}^{(\mathbf{n})}$ and boundary micro-tractions $\hat{\mathbf{q}}_\alpha^{(\mathbf{n})}$. The macro-forces act on the degrees of freedom in $\mathbf{u}$, whereas the micro-forces act on the degrees of freedom in $\mathbf{a}_\alpha$. It is possible to define additional external force descriptions, the reader is referred to [74, 90]. The external virtual work $\mathcal{W}_{ext}$ in the Lagrangian form, integrating the external forces over $\mathcal{S}$ and $\partial\mathcal{S}_N$, is defined as follows

$$\mathcal{W}_{ext}\,(\mathbf{u},\mathbf{w}) = \int_{\mathcal{B}} \mathbf{b}\cdot\delta\mathbf{u}\;dV + \int_{\mathcal{B}} \mathbf{l}_\alpha\cdot\delta\mathbf{w}_\alpha\;dV + \int_{\partial\mathcal{B}_N} \hat{\mathbf{t}}^{(\mathbf{n})}\cdot\delta\mathbf{u}\;dA + \int_{\partial\mathcal{B}_N} \hat{\mathbf{q}}_\alpha^{(\mathbf{n})}\cdot\delta\mathbf{w}_\alpha\;dA \tag{4.48}$$

The first law of thermodynamics with balance of mechanical energy, where $\ddot{\mathbf{u}} = 0$, provides the following variational principle

$$\delta\tilde{\Psi}(\mathbf{u},\mathbf{w}) - \mathcal{W}_{ext} = \frac{1}{2}\int_{\mathcal{B}}\int_{\mathcal{S}} \left\{\tilde{\mathbf{S}}^{(0)} : \delta\tilde{\mathbf{C}}^{(0)} + \tilde{\mathbf{S}}^{(1)} : \delta\tilde{\mathbf{C}}^{(1)} + \tilde{\mathbf{S}}^{(2)} : \delta\tilde{\mathbf{C}}^{(2)}\right\} dS\,dV - \mathcal{W}_{ext} = 0. \tag{4.49}$$

The governing equations of the micromorphic variational principle (Eq. (4.49)) are found by substituting $\delta\tilde{\mathbf{C}} = \delta\mathbf{C} + \zeta^\alpha\delta\mathbf{K}_\alpha$ from Eq. (4.30)-(4.34), and expressed using index notation and to a curvilinear coordinate system, to give

$$\begin{aligned}\int_{\mathcal{B}}\int_{\mathcal{S}} \frac{1}{2}\Big\{\; & \tilde{S}_{ij}^{(0)}\,\tilde{\mathbf{G}}^i\otimes\tilde{\mathbf{G}}^j : \left(\delta C_{kl}^{(0)}\,\tilde{\mathbf{G}}^k\otimes\tilde{\mathbf{G}}^l + \zeta^\alpha\delta K_{kl}^{(0)\alpha}\,\tilde{\mathbf{G}}^k\otimes\tilde{\mathbf{G}}^l\right)\\ + \; & \tilde{S}_{i\beta}^{(1)}\left(\tilde{\mathbf{G}}^i\otimes\tilde{\mathbf{I}}^\beta + \tilde{\mathbf{I}}^\beta\otimes\tilde{\mathbf{G}}^i\right) : [\delta C_{j\gamma}^{(1)} + \zeta^\alpha\delta K_{j\gamma}^{(1)\alpha}]\left(\tilde{\mathbf{G}}^j\otimes\tilde{\mathbf{I}}^\gamma + \tilde{\mathbf{I}}^\gamma\otimes\tilde{\mathbf{G}}^j\right)\\ + \; & \tilde{S}_{\beta\gamma}^{(2)}\,\tilde{\mathbf{I}}^\beta\otimes\tilde{\mathbf{I}}^\gamma : \left(\delta C_{\lambda\mu}^{(2)}\,\tilde{\mathbf{I}}^\lambda\otimes\tilde{\mathbf{I}}^\mu + \zeta^\alpha\delta K_{\lambda\mu}^{(2)\alpha}\,\tilde{\mathbf{I}}^\lambda\otimes\tilde{\mathbf{I}}^\mu\right)\Big\}\,dS\,dV - \mathcal{W}_{ext} = 0.\end{aligned} \tag{4.50}$$

Further, we integrate over the micro-space $\mathcal{S}$ to get homogenized stresses ($\tilde{\mathbf{S}} \to \mathbf{S}$) using the conversion metrics $\tilde{G}^{tv} = \tilde{\mathbf{G}}^t\cdot\tilde{\mathbf{G}}^v$ and $\tilde{I}^{\alpha\beta} = \tilde{\mathbf{I}}^\alpha\cdot\tilde{\mathbf{I}}^\beta$ to account for the double contraction of the basis vectors, as follows

$$S^{(0)vw} = \int_{\mathcal{S}} \tilde{S}_{rt}^{(0)}\tilde{G}^{rv}\,\tilde{G}^{tw}\,dS; \quad S^{(1)k\gamma} = \int_{\mathcal{S}} 4\,\tilde{S}_{r\beta}^{(1)}\tilde{G}^{rk}\,\tilde{I}^{\beta\gamma}\,dS; \quad S^{(2)\lambda\mu} = \int_{\mathcal{S}} \tilde{S}_{\beta\gamma}^{(2)}\tilde{I}^{\beta\lambda}\,\tilde{I}^{\gamma\mu}\,dS, \tag{4.51}$$

and homogenize the higher-order stress terms, notated by $\zeta^\alpha\tilde{\mathbf{S}} \to \mathbf{M}^\alpha$, as follows

$$M^{(0)\alpha,vw} = \int_{\mathcal{S}} \zeta^\alpha\tilde{S}_{rt}^{(0)}\tilde{G}^{rv}\,\tilde{G}^{tw}\,dS; \quad M^{(1)\alpha,k\gamma} = \int_{\mathcal{S}} 4\,\zeta^\alpha\tilde{S}_{r\beta}^{(1)}\tilde{G}^{rk}\,\tilde{I}^{\beta\gamma}\,dS; \quad M^{(2)\alpha,\lambda\mu} = \int_{\mathcal{S}} \zeta^\alpha\tilde{S}_{\beta\gamma}^{(2)}\tilde{I}^{\beta\lambda}\,\tilde{I}^{\gamma\mu}\,dS, \tag{4.52}$$

whereby all of the mixed-scale basis vectors double contractions are treated as complementary, and hence we find $4\,\tilde{G}^{rk}\,\tilde{I}^{\beta\gamma}$ in Eq. (4.51)-(4.52). The integration over the micro-space $\mathcal{S}$ provides that the micro-structure characterizing internal length scale parameters $l_\alpha$ associated with the different dimensions of $\mathcal{S}$ are implicitly incorporated, such that the coordinates of the micro-space $\zeta^\alpha$ are defined over the intervals $[-\frac{l_\alpha}{2}; \frac{l_\alpha}{2}]$. It is worth noting that the conversion metrics are not required if stress tensors with contravariant basis vectors $\tilde{\mathbf{G}}_t$ and $\tilde{\mathbf{I}}_\alpha$ are used instead in the variational formulation, as the resulting contraction with the covariant basis vectors of the strain tensors would produce a *Kronecker* delta, i.e. $\tilde{\mathbf{G}}_t \otimes \tilde{\mathbf{G}}^v = \delta_t^{\ v}$; however, this was not implemented in this study. We now substitute the homogenized stresses of Eq. (4.51)-(4.52) and the strain measures variants from Appendix A.1.1 into Eq. (4.50) to arrive at

$$\begin{aligned}\int_{\mathcal{B}} \frac{1}{2}\Big\{ & S^{(0)kl}\left(F_{rl}\,\delta u_{r,k} + F_{rk}\,\delta u_{r,l}\right) + M^{(0)\alpha,kl}\left(\delta a_{\alpha r,k} F_{rl} + a_{\alpha r,k}\delta u_{r,l} + \delta a_{\alpha r,l} F_{rk} + a_{\alpha r,l}\delta u_{r,k}\right)\\ &+ S^{(1)j\gamma}\left(a_{\gamma r}\delta u_{r,j} + F_{rj}\delta a_{\gamma r}\right) + M^{(1)\alpha,j\gamma}\left(\delta a_{\alpha r,j} a_{\gamma r} + a_{\alpha r,j}\delta a_{\gamma r}\right)\\ &+ S^{(2)\lambda\mu}\left(\delta a_{\lambda r} a_{\mu r} + a_{\lambda r}\delta a_{\mu r}\right)\Big\} dV - \mathcal{W}_{ext} = 0.\end{aligned} \tag{4.53}$$

We can then apply *Gauss'* divergence theorem in the Cartesian frame ($\tilde{\mathbf{G}}^i = \tilde{\mathbf{G}}^i = \mathbf{e}_i$) and assume $\delta\mathbf{u} = 0$ and $\delta\mathbf{w}_\alpha = 0$ on $\partial\mathcal{B}_D$ to give

$$\begin{aligned}&\int_{\mathcal{B}} \frac{1}{2}\Big\{ -\frac{\partial}{\partial\vartheta^k} S^{(0)kl} F_{rl}\delta u_r - \frac{\partial}{\partial\vartheta^l} S^{(0)kl} F_{rk}\delta u_r - \frac{\partial}{\partial\vartheta^j} S^{(1)j\gamma} a_{\gamma r}\delta u_r\\ &\qquad - \frac{\partial}{\partial\vartheta^l} M^{(0)\alpha,kl} a_{\alpha r,k}\delta u_r - \frac{\partial}{\partial\vartheta^k} M^{(0)\alpha,kl} a_{\alpha r,l}\delta u_r - b_r\delta u_r \Big\} dV\\ &+ \int_{\mathcal{B}} \frac{1}{2}\Big\{ S^{(1)j\gamma} F_{rj}\delta a_{\gamma r} + S^{(2)\lambda\mu} a_{\mu r}\delta a_{\lambda r} + S^{(2)\lambda\mu} a_{\lambda r}\delta a_{\mu r}\\ &\qquad - \frac{\partial}{\partial\vartheta^k} M^{(0)\alpha,kl} F_{rl}\delta a_{\alpha r} - \frac{\partial}{\partial\vartheta^l} M^{(0)\alpha,kl} F_{rk}\delta a_{\alpha r}\\ &\qquad - \frac{\partial}{\partial\vartheta^j} M^{(1)\alpha,j\gamma} a_{\gamma r}\delta a_{\alpha r} - M^{(1)\alpha,j\gamma} a_{\alpha r,j}\delta a_{\gamma r} - l_{\alpha r}\delta a_{\alpha r} \Big\} dV\\ &+ \int_{\partial\mathcal{B}_N} \frac{1}{2}\Big\{ S^{(0)kl} F_{rl} n_k\delta u_r + S^{(0)kl} F_{rk} n_l\delta u_r + S^{(1)j\gamma} a_{\gamma r} n_j\delta u_r\\ &\qquad + M^{(0)\alpha,kl} a_{\alpha r,k} n_l\delta u_r + M^{(0)\alpha,kl} a_{\alpha r,l} n_k\delta u_r - \hat{t}_r^{(n)}\delta u_r \Big\} dA,\\ &+ \int_{\partial\mathcal{B}_N} \frac{1}{2}\Big\{ M^{(0)\alpha,kl} F_{rl} n_k\delta a_{\alpha r} + M^{(0)\alpha,kl} F_{rk} n_l\delta a_{\alpha r}\\ &\qquad + M^{(1)\alpha,j\gamma} a_{\gamma r} n_j\delta a_{\alpha r} - \hat{q}_{\alpha r}^{(\mathbf{n})}\delta a_{\alpha r} \Big\} dA.\end{aligned} \tag{4.54}$$

Taking into account $\delta\mathbf{u}$ is a free variation and $\delta\mathbf{a}_\alpha$ is a free variation, and ensuring all variants $\delta\mathbf{a}$ have the same index $\alpha$, we identify the following equilibrium equations [74, 90] in and on the macro-space

$$\begin{aligned}&- \frac{\partial}{\partial\vartheta^k} S^{(0)kl} F_{rl} - \frac{\partial}{\partial\vartheta^l} S^{(0)kl} F_{rk} - \frac{\partial}{\partial\vartheta^j} S^{(1)j\gamma} a_{\gamma r}\\ &- \frac{\partial}{\partial\vartheta^l} M^{(0)\alpha,kl} a_{\alpha r,k} - \frac{\partial}{\partial\vartheta^k} M^{(0)\alpha,kl} a_{\alpha r,l} - b_r = 0 \quad \text{in } \mathcal{B}\end{aligned} \tag{4.55}$$

$$\begin{aligned}&S^{(1)j\alpha} F_{rj} + S^{(2)\alpha\mu} a_{\mu r} + S^{(2)\lambda\alpha} a_{\lambda r}\\ &- \frac{\partial}{\partial\vartheta^k} M^{(0)\alpha,kl} F_{rl} - \frac{\partial}{\partial\vartheta^l} M^{(0)\alpha,kl} F_{rk}\\ &- \frac{\partial}{\partial\vartheta^j} M^{(1)\alpha,j\gamma} a_{\gamma r} + M^{(1)\beta,j\alpha} a_{\beta r,j} - l_{\alpha r} = 0 \quad \text{in } \mathcal{B}\end{aligned} \tag{4.56}$$

and corresponding *Neumann* boundaries

$$\begin{aligned}&S^{(0)kl} F_{rl} n_k + S^{(0)kl} F_{rk} n_l + S^{(1)j\gamma} a_{\gamma r} n_j\\ &+ M^{(0)\alpha,kl} a_{\alpha r,k} n_l + M^{(0)\alpha,kl} a_{\alpha r,l} n_k - \hat{t}_r^{(\mathbf{n})} = 0 \quad \text{on } \partial\mathcal{B}_N\end{aligned} \tag{4.57}$$

$$M^{(0)\alpha,kl}\,F_{rl}n_k + M^{(0)\alpha,kl}\,F_{rk}n_l + M^{(1)\alpha,j\gamma}\,a_{\gamma r}n_j - \hat{q}^{(\mathbf{n})}_{\alpha r} = 0 \quad \text{on } \partial\mathcal{B}_N. \tag{4.58}$$

The linearization of $\tilde{\Psi}(\mathbf{u},\mathbf{w})$ is found in Appendix A.2.1.

### 4.3.2 MDO micromorphic model variational formulation

The variational formulation for the MDO micromorphic model continues from Eq. (4.49) as follows

$$\delta\breve{\Psi}(\mathbf{u},\mathbf{w}) - \mathcal{W}_{ext} = \frac{1}{2}\int_{\mathcal{B}}\left\{\breve{\mathbf{S}}^{(0)} : \delta\breve{\mathbf{C}}^{(0)} + \varsigma^{\alpha}\breve{\mathbf{S}}^{(1)} : \delta\breve{\mathbf{C}}^{(1)}_{\alpha} + \varsigma^{\alpha}\varsigma^{\beta}\breve{\mathbf{S}}^{(2)} : \delta\breve{\mathbf{C}}^{(2)}_{\alpha\beta}\right\} dV - \mathcal{W}_{ext} = 0, \tag{4.59}$$

where $\mathcal{W}_{ext}$ is defined as per Eq. (4.48). We then substitute the MDO strain measures variants from Appendix A.1.2, and the conversion metrics for the basis vector contraction is accounted for with $\breve{G}^{tv} = \breve{\mathbf{G}}^t \cdot \breve{\mathbf{G}}^v = \delta^{tv}$, because the simple case $\breve{\mathbf{G}}^t = \mathbf{e}_t$ of Eq. (4.40) is used for this study. Thus we find

$$\begin{aligned}
\frac{1}{2}\int_{\mathcal{B}}\Big\{\; & \breve{S}^{(0)kl}\left(F_{rl}\,\delta u_{r,k} + F_{rk}\,\delta u_{r,l}\right) \\
+\; & \varsigma^{\alpha}\breve{S}^{(1)kl}\left(\delta a_{\alpha r,k}F_{rl} + a_{\alpha r,k}\delta u_{r,l} + \delta a_{\alpha r,l}F_{rk} + a_{\alpha r,l}\delta u_{r,k}\right) \\
+\; & \varsigma^{\alpha}\varsigma^{\beta}\breve{S}^{(2)kl}\left[\delta a_{\alpha r,k}a_{\beta r,l} + a_{\alpha r,k}\delta a_{\beta r,l}\right]\Big\}\, dV - \mathcal{W}_{ext} = 0.
\end{aligned} \tag{4.60}$$

We can then apply *Gauss*' divergence theorem in the Cartesian frame ($\breve{\mathbf{G}}^i = \breve{\mathbf{G}}^i = \mathbf{e}_i$) and assume $\delta\mathbf{u} = 0$ and $\delta\mathbf{w}_\alpha = 0$ on $\partial\mathcal{B}_D$ to give

$$\begin{aligned}
&\int_{\mathcal{B}}\frac{1}{2}\Big\{ -\frac{\partial}{\partial\vartheta^k}\,\breve{S}^{(0)kl}\,F_{rl}\delta u_r - \frac{\partial}{\partial\vartheta^l}\,\breve{S}^{(0)kl}F_{rk}\delta u_r \\
&\qquad -\frac{\partial}{\partial\vartheta^l}\varsigma^{\alpha}\breve{S}^{(1)kl}\,a_{\alpha r,k}\delta u_r - \frac{\partial}{\partial\vartheta^k}\varsigma^{\alpha}\breve{S}^{(1)kl}\,a_{\alpha r,l}\delta u_r - b_r\delta u_r\Big\}dV \\
&\int_{\mathcal{B}}\frac{1}{2}\Big\{ -\frac{\partial}{\partial\vartheta^k}\varsigma^{\alpha}\breve{S}^{(1)kl}F_{rl}\delta a_{\alpha r} - \frac{\partial}{\partial\vartheta^l}\varsigma^{\alpha}\breve{S}^{(1)kl}F_{rk}\delta a_{\alpha r} \\
&\qquad -\frac{\partial}{\partial\vartheta^k}\varsigma^{\alpha}\varsigma^{\beta}\breve{S}^{(2)kl}a_{\beta r,l}\delta a_{\alpha r} - \frac{\partial}{\partial\vartheta^l}\varsigma^{\alpha}\varsigma^{\beta}\breve{S}^{(2)kl}a_{\alpha r,k}\delta a_{\beta r} - l_{\alpha r}\delta a_{\alpha r}\Big\}dV \\
&+\int_{\partial\mathcal{B}_N}\frac{1}{2}\Big\{ \breve{S}^{(0)kl}\,F_{rl}n_k\delta u_r + \breve{S}^{(0)kl}F_{rk}n_l\delta u_r \\
&\qquad +\varsigma^{\alpha}\breve{S}^{(1)kl}\,a_{\alpha r,k}n_l\delta u_r + \varsigma^{\alpha}\breve{S}^{(1)kl}\,a_{\alpha r,l}n_k\delta u_r - \hat{t}^{(\mathbf{n})}_r\delta u_r\Big\}dA \\
&+\int_{\partial\mathcal{B}_N}\frac{1}{2}\Big\{ \varsigma^{\alpha}\breve{S}^{(1)kl}F_{rl}n_k\delta a_{\alpha r} + \varsigma^{\alpha}\breve{S}^{(1)kl}F_{rk}n_l\delta a_{\alpha r} \\
&\qquad +\varsigma^{\alpha}\varsigma^{\beta}\breve{S}^{(2)kl}a_{\beta r,l}n_k\delta a_{\alpha r} + \varsigma^{\alpha}\varsigma^{\beta}\breve{S}^{(2)kl}a_{\alpha r,k}n_l\delta a_{\beta r} - \hat{q}^{(\mathbf{n})}_{\alpha r}\delta a_{\alpha r}\Big\}dA.
\end{aligned} \tag{4.61}$$

Taking into account $\delta\mathbf{u}$ is a free variation and $\delta\mathbf{a}_\alpha$ is a free variation, and ensuring all variants $\delta\mathbf{a}$ have the same index $\alpha$, we identify the following equilibrium equations in and on the macro-space

$$\begin{aligned}
&-\frac{\partial}{\partial\vartheta^k}\,\breve{S}^{(0)kl}\,F_{rl} - \frac{\partial}{\partial\vartheta^l}\,\breve{S}^{(0)kl}F_{rk} \\
&-\frac{\partial}{\partial\vartheta^l}\varsigma^{\alpha}\breve{S}^{(1)kl}\,a_{\alpha r,k} - \frac{\partial}{\partial\vartheta^k}\varsigma^{\alpha}\breve{S}^{(1)kl}\,a_{\alpha r,l} - b_r = 0 \quad \text{in } \mathcal{B}
\end{aligned} \tag{4.62}$$

$$\begin{aligned}
&-\frac{\partial}{\partial\vartheta^k}\varsigma^{\alpha}\breve{S}^{(1)kl}F_{rl} - \frac{\partial}{\partial\vartheta^l}\varsigma^{\alpha}\breve{S}^{(1)kl}F_{rk} \\
&-\frac{\partial}{\partial\vartheta^k}\varsigma^{\alpha}\varsigma^{\beta}\breve{S}^{(2)kl}a_{\beta r,l} - \frac{\partial}{\partial\vartheta^l}\varsigma^{\alpha}\varsigma^{\beta}\breve{S}^{(2)kl}a_{\beta r,k} - l_{\alpha r} = 0 \quad \text{in } \mathcal{B}
\end{aligned} \tag{4.63}$$

and corresponding *Neumann* boundaries

$$\breve{S}^{(0)kl}\,F_{rl}n_k + \breve{S}^{(0)kl}F_{rk}n_l + \zeta^\alpha \breve{S}^{(1)kl}\,a_{\alpha r,k}n_l + \zeta^\alpha \breve{S}^{(1)kl}\,a_{\alpha r,l}n_k - \hat{t}_r^{(\mathbf{n})} = 0 \quad \text{on } \partial\mathcal{B}_N \tag{4.64}$$

$$\zeta^\alpha \breve{S}^{(1)kl}F_{rl}n_k + \zeta^\alpha \breve{S}^{(1)kl}F_{rk}n_l + \zeta^\alpha\zeta^\beta \breve{S}^{(2)kl}a_{\beta r,l}n_k + \zeta^\alpha\zeta^\beta \breve{S}^{(2)kl}a_{\beta r,k}n_l - \hat{q}_{\alpha r}^{(\mathbf{n})} = 0 \quad \text{on } \partial\mathcal{B}_N. \tag{4.65}$$

The linearization of $\breve{\Psi}(\mathbf{u},\mathbf{w})$ is found in Appendix A.2.2.

## 4.4 Micromorphic constitutive model

The micromorphic model has additional strain measures over classical models, which increases the ability of the model to replicate material behaviour as originated in the underlying micro-structure. The stress responses to these additional strain measures are described by extra constitutive equations. The micromorphic model has three scales of stress and strain measures $(\tilde{\mathbf{S}}^{(i)}, \tilde{\mathbf{C}}^{(i)}, \tilde{\mathbf{E}}^{(i)})$, and hence three separate strain energy functions $(\tilde{\psi}^{(i)})$: the macro-scale $(\tilde{\mathbf{S}}^{(0)}, \tilde{\mathbf{C}}^{(0)}, \tilde{\mathbf{E}}^{(0)}, \tilde{\psi}^{(0)})$ which are the same as the classical stress and strain measures $(\mathbf{S}, \mathbf{C}, \mathbf{E})$; the mixed-scale $(\tilde{\mathbf{S}}^{(1)}, \tilde{\mathbf{C}}^{(1)}, \tilde{\mathbf{E}}^{(1)}, \tilde{\psi}^{(1)})$; and the micro-scale $(\tilde{\mathbf{S}}^{(2)}, \tilde{\mathbf{C}}^{(2)}, \tilde{\mathbf{E}}^{(2)}, \tilde{\psi}^{(2)})$. This study makes use of a micromorphic continuum with only one micro-dimension/micro-director.

### 4.4.1 Macro-scale constitutive law

Section 3.5 motivated why there is a need to use orthotropic constitutive law to model the complex deformations of cardiac tissue, and the additional micromorphic contributions can notably enrich the orthotropy. However, in the process of validating and calibrating the micromorphic model both macro-scale isotropy and orthotropy was used, as well as linear and nonlinear constitutive laws.

#### 4.4.1.1 Isotropic macro-scale

In order to better understand the influence of the micromorphic mixed-scale $\tilde{\psi}^{(1)}$ and micro-scale $\tilde{\psi}^{(2)}$ strain energy function contributions and their material parameters, it is most transparent to use an isotropic constitutive law for the macro-scale strain energy $\tilde{\psi}^{(0)}$. A material is deemed isotropic if its mechanical properties can be described without reference to directions [48], and thus any anisotropic behaviour must then be attributed to the micromorphic mixed-scale and micro-scale contributions, which allows for clear analysis of the mixed-scale and micro-scale material parameter effects. The isotropic macro-scale constitutive law used in the numerical examples of Section 5 is based on an isotropic linear elastic material, which is defined by the strain energy function

$$\tilde{\psi}^{(0)}\left(\tilde{\mathbf{E}}^{(0)}\right) = \frac{1}{2}b_0 \operatorname{tr}\left(\tilde{\mathbf{E}}^{(0)}\right)^2 + \frac{1}{2}a_0 \operatorname{tr}\left((\tilde{\mathbf{E}}^{(0)})^2\right). \tag{4.66}$$

It is worth noting that, in conjunction with an isotropic macro-scale, the micromorphic micro-scale contributions create a preferred material direction along the micro-fibre axis, and thus the overall material law is in fact transversely isotropic.

#### 4.4.1.2 Orthotropic macro-scale

The motivation for using orthotropic constitutive law to model cardiac tissue was previously given in Section 2.5 and Section 3.5. It is possible to create an orthotropic model from the anisotropic contributions of the mixed-scale and micro-scale only. This can be achieved most effectively by using two or more micro-directors with differing material parameters. Alternatively for the simplest case of one micro-director, the mixed-scale shearing $\tilde{\mathbf{C}}^{(1)}$ of the bulk material against the micro-directors has components in orthogonal directions, and each component can have a unique material parameter, thus resulting in an orthotropic response. The intended use of the micromorphic model is to interpret its micro-directors as the muscle fibres in cardiac tissue, and the macro-scale would represent the ECM holding the muscle fibres in place. However, the review of the contributions of the myocardium by Fomovsky et al. (2010) highlights clear characteristic responses from the myocytes and the ECM. In particular, the ECM exhibits significant nonlinearity coupled with directional dependency, and thus in order for the macro-scale to represent the ECM accurately it would need have a nonlinear, orthotropic constitutive law.

The ECM accounts for the majority of the stiffness of myocardial tissue at large strains, and thus the same constitutive law for the classical model of Usyk et al. (2002) in Section 3.5 will be used for the macro-scale of the micromorphic model, but with new material parameters to allow for the mixed-scale and micro-scale contributions. Although the micro-directors representing muscle fibres will make a smaller contribution to the tissue's passive mechanics, the micro-directors will play a pivotal role in future studies where the active stress of contracting muscle fibres can be implemented through the micro-directors. Following on from Section 3.5, the three orthonormal material covariant directions of myocardial tissue - namely the muscle fibres $\mathbf{V}_f$, sheet $\mathbf{V}_s$ and sheet-normal $\mathbf{V}_n$ - can form the bases of a micromorphic *Green* 'fibre' strain tensor associated with the orthonormal basis $(\mathbf{V}_f, \mathbf{V}_s, \mathbf{V}_n)$ such that

$$\begin{aligned}\tilde{\mathbf{E}}^{(0)} = {} & \tilde{E}^{(0)}_{ff}\mathbf{V}^f \otimes \mathbf{V}^f + \tilde{E}^{(0)}_{ss}\mathbf{V}^s \otimes \mathbf{V}^s + \tilde{E}^{(0)}_{nn}\mathbf{V}^n \otimes \mathbf{V}^n + \tilde{E}^{(0)}_{fs}\left(\mathbf{V}^f \otimes \mathbf{V}^s + \mathbf{V}^s \otimes \mathbf{V}^f\right) \\ & + \tilde{E}^{(0)}_{fn}\left(\mathbf{V}^f \otimes \mathbf{V}^n + \mathbf{V}^n \otimes \mathbf{V}^f\right) + \tilde{E}^{(0)}_{sn}\left(\mathbf{V}^s \otimes \mathbf{V}^n + \mathbf{V}^n \otimes \mathbf{V}^s\right),\end{aligned} \tag{4.67}$$

where the macro-scale strain $\tilde{\mathbf{E}}^{(0)}$ notation has replaced the classical strain $\mathbf{E}$ notation of Eq. (3.26). Similarly, the classical strain energy function used by Usyk et al. (2000) to formulate the left ventricular passive filling constitutive is adapted for the micromorphic model $\tilde{\psi}^{(0)}_{\text{pass.}}$, where the orthotropy and non-linearity is contained in $\tilde{\psi}^{(0)}_{\text{orth./exp.}}$, as well as the near incompressibility in $\tilde{\psi}^{(0)}_{\text{comp.}}$:

$$\tilde{\psi}^{(0)}_{\text{pass.}} = \tilde{\psi}^{(0)}_{\text{orth./exp.}} + \tilde{\psi}^{(0)}_{\text{comp.}} = \frac{1}{2}A_0\left(e^{Q^{(0)}} - 1\right) + A_{\text{comp}}\left[J\,ln(J) - J + 1\right], \tag{4.68}$$

where

$$\begin{aligned}Q^{(0)} = {} & b_{ff}(\tilde{E}^{(0)}_{ff})^2 + b_{ss}(\tilde{E}^{(0)}_{ss})^2 + b_{nn}(\tilde{E}^{(0)}_{nn})^2 \\ & + b_{fs}\left((\tilde{E}^{(0)}_{fs})^2 + (\tilde{E}^{(0)}_{sf})^2\right) + b_{fn}\left((\tilde{E}^{(0)}_{fn})^2 + (\tilde{E}^{(0)}_{nf})^2\right) + b_{sn}\left((\tilde{E}^{(0)}_{sn})^2 + (\tilde{E}^{(0)}_{ns})^2\right).\end{aligned} \tag{4.69}$$

In Eq. (4.69) the material parameters $b_{ij}$ determine the material anisotropy, and in Eq. (4.68) $J$ is the Jacobian, the parameter $A_0$ is used as a global stress scaling coefficient, and $A_{\text{comp}}$ is the compressibility coefficient. For details on an invariant based approach for this constitutive law, refer to Section 3.5.

### 4.4.2 Mixed-scale and micro-scale constitutive law

The mixed-scale and micro-scale are given strain energy functions that produce linear material behaviour for the numerical examples of Section 5, as well as strain energy functions that produce non-linear material behaviour for the cardiac models of Section 6. The micromorphic mixed-scale and micro-scale *Green* 'fibre' strain tensors are defined for single micro-director orientated with the muscle fibres $\mathbf{V}_f$, as done in Eq. (4.67), to give

$$\tilde{\mathbf{E}}^{(1)} = \tilde{E}^{(1)}_{ff}\mathbf{V}^f \otimes \mathbf{V}^f + \tilde{E}^{(1)}_{sf}\left(\mathbf{V}^f \otimes \mathbf{V}^s + \mathbf{V}^s \otimes \mathbf{V}^f\right) + \tilde{E}^{(1)}_{nf}\left(\mathbf{V}^f \otimes \mathbf{V}^n + \mathbf{V}^n \otimes \mathbf{V}^f\right) \tag{4.70}$$

$$\tilde{\mathbf{E}}^{(2)} = \tilde{E}^{(2)}_{ff}\mathbf{V}^f \otimes \mathbf{V}^f, \tag{4.71}$$

where the shearing $\tilde{\mathbf{E}}^{(1)}$ of the muscle fibre with the ECM can occur in all three characteristic directions of the cardiac tissue $(\mathbf{V}_f, \mathbf{V}_s, \mathbf{V}_n)$, whereas the fibre strain $\tilde{\mathbf{E}}^{(2)}$ can only experience strain along its axis $(\mathbf{V}_f)$. We breakdown the strain energy functions with $\tilde{\psi}^{(1)}(Q^{(1)})$ and $\tilde{\psi}^{(2)}(Q^{(2)})$ such that

$$Q^{(1)} = \left(\tilde{E}^{(1)}_{ff}\right)^2 + \left(\tilde{E}^{(1)}_{sf}\right)^2 + \left(\tilde{E}^{(1)}_{nf}\right)^2, \quad \text{and} \quad Q^{(2)} = \left(\tilde{E}^{(2)}_{ff}\right)^2. \tag{4.72}$$

#### 4.4.2.1 Linear material behaviour from mixed-scale and micro-scale

In the case of the numerical examples of Section 5, it is more transparent to use a linear material response from the mixed-scale and micro-scale to determine the respective behaviour of the scales, and as such the mixed-scale $\tilde{\psi}^{(1)}$ and micro-scale $\tilde{\psi}^{(2)}$ strain energy functions are

$$\tilde{\psi}^{(1)} = \frac{1}{2}A_1 Q^{(1)}, \quad \text{and} \quad \tilde{\psi}^{(2)} = \frac{1}{2}A_2 Q^{(2)}. \tag{4.73}$$

#### 4.4.2.2 Non-linear material behaviour from mixed-scale and micro-scale

Muscle fibres will exhibit non-linear behaviour, as is common with biological tissues. It is therefore useful to cast the mixed-scale and the micro-scale strain energy functions into an exponential function as follows

$$\tilde{\psi}^{(1)} = \frac{1}{2}A_1\left(e^{(B_1 Q^{(1)})} - 1\right), \quad \text{and} \quad \tilde{\psi}^{(2)} = \frac{1}{2}A_2\left(e^{(B_2 Q^{(2)})} - 1\right). \tag{4.74}$$

Now that the kinematics, variational principles and constitutive models for both Sansour's model and the MDO model have been set out, the fundamental behaviour of the micromorphic models is assessed in the numerical examples of Section 5.

5

# Numerical Examples

The intent of this research is to apply a micromorphic continuum model to simulating cardiac tissue. However, before launching into complex non-linear, orthotropic heart models with patient-specific geometries, it is important to get a better understanding of the micromorphic model's characteristics on clearer and more discernible numerical examples. For classical continuum models, it is more straightforward to identify the parts of the mathematical formulation that dictate the material response to the various strain modes. However, the micromorphic model has three strain-scales with their own strain measures that make overlapping contributions to the material response. The isotropic strain energy function of Eq. (4.66) in Section 4.4 producing a linear material response for the macro-scale $\tilde{\psi}^{(0)}$ was used in this section so that any anisotropic material response could be attributed to the micromorphic mixed-scale and micro-scale contributions. Similarly, the strain energy functions in Eq. (4.73) producing a linear material response for the mixed-scale $\tilde{\psi}^{(1)}$ and micro-scale $\tilde{\psi}^{(2)}$ were used in this chapter to best interpret the influence of these scales. The effect of the mixed-scale and micro-scale material parameters on the micro-director deformation, uniqueness of solutions, and strain-dependent anisotropy are some of the properties investigated in this section through numerical examples such as a simple tension beam or a perforated plate under biaxial tension.

## 5.1 Mixed-scale and micro-scale material parameter influence

Preliminary testing of Sansour's micromorphic model revealed two important characteristics of the model: the model cannot be solved for certain mixed-scale and micro-scale material parameter combinations; and whether the micro-director stretches or contracts can also depend on the mixed-scale and micro-scale parameter combinations. Both scenarios can be explained using the energy balances we derived in Section 4.3; the energy balance over the macro-scale displacement degrees of freedom ($\mathbf{u}$) in Eq. (4.55), and the energy balance over the micro-scale displacement degrees of freedom ($\mathbf{a}_\alpha$) in Eq. (4.56). For the following scenario: in the absence of body forces; ignoring higher-order terms ($l_\alpha \ll 1$); exploiting the symmetry of $\mathbf{S}^{(2)}$; and extracting the factor 4 absorbed into Eq. (4.51), we find the energy balance of Eq. (4.56) becomes

$$4\,S^{(1)j\gamma}F_{rj} + 2\,S^{(2)\gamma\mu}a_{\mu r} = 0 \tag{5.1}$$

$$\therefore\ 2\,S^{(1)j\gamma}F_{rj} = -S^{(2)\gamma\mu}a_{\mu r}. \tag{5.2}$$

It must be noted that Eq. (5.2) is dependent on the interpretation chosen for the double contraction of the mixed-scale basis vectors in Eq. (4.51), whereby this study used a factor 4 as previously mentioned in Section 4.3.1. The significance of the relationship shown in Eq. (5.2) will be explained in the following sections.

### 5.1.1 Proof for unsolvable model scenario

It was uncovered in this study that there are scenarios where the micromorphic model does not have a unique solution, and thus the model cannot be solved. This phenomenon is caused by the material parameters of the mixed-scale and micro-scale. The author devised the following novel proof to explain the cause of this problem. Let us examine a simple tension beam subjected to homogeneous deformation with the beam's axis aligned along the x-axis, as well as the undeformed micro-director aligned along the x-axis ($\mathbf{a}^0_\gamma = \mathbf{e}_1$, where $\gamma = 1$), as seen in Figure 5.1.

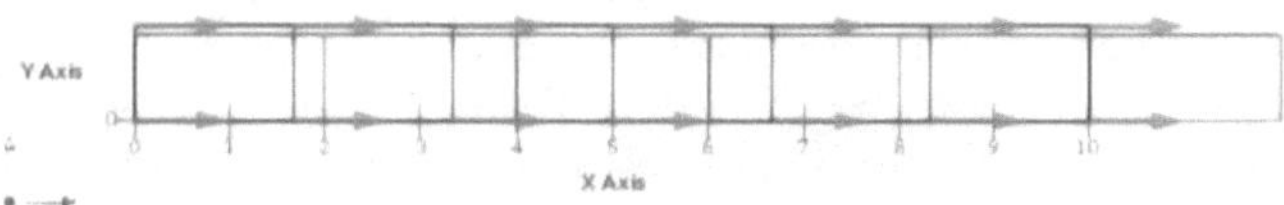


Fig. 5.1: Homogeneous deformation tension beam example: undeformed beam seen in black; deformed beam seen in red for $\bar{u}_{(E)1} = 2$ m; and initial micro-director orientation seen in green ($\mathbf{a}^0_\gamma = \mathbf{e}_1$). A large prescribed displacement was chosen for this figure to emphasize the homogeneous deformation.

It is possible to include all the constituent terms with known values into Eq. (5.2), in order to solve for the micro-director deformation or a material parameter as desired. Since the mixed-scale and micro-scale stress terms in this example are derived from the strain energy functions of Eq. (4.73), the stress terms can be divided into the corresponding mixed-scale ($A_1$) and micro-scale ($A_2$) material parameters, and *Green* strain measures, given that $\mathbf{S}^{(i)} \propto A_i \mathbf{E}^{(i)}$, and hence Eq. (5.2) becomes

$$2\,A_1 E^{(1)j\gamma} F_{rj} = -A_2 E^{(2)\gamma\mu} a_{\mu r}. \tag{5.3}$$

Furthermore, the equation can be represented in terms of the right *Cauchy-Green* strains using the fact that $\mathbf{E}^{(i)} = 1/2(\mathbf{C}^{(i)} - \mathbf{C}^{(i)0})$, and thus

$$2\,A_1 \left(C^{(1)j\gamma} - C^{(1)0j\gamma}\right) F_{rj} = -A_2 \left(C^{(2)\gamma\mu} - C^{(2)0\gamma\mu}\right) a_{\mu r}. \tag{5.4}$$

We substitute the deformation terms of the right *Cauchy-Green* strains of Eq. (4.31) and Eq. (4.32) to give

$$2\,A_1 \left(x_{s,j} a_{\gamma s} - \delta_{sj} a^0_{\gamma s}\right) F_{rj} = -A_2 \left(a_{\gamma s} a_{\mu s} - a^0_{\gamma s} a^0_{\mu s}\right) a_{\mu r}. \tag{5.5}$$

This deformation-driven tension beam example is slender enough to ignore the effects of transverse contraction, therefore the stretch $\lambda$ of the macro-scale simplifies to $\lambda = F_{11}$ , and we found from the simulation that $F_{22} \approx F_{33} \approx 1$. Similarly, it was confirmed in simulations that the micro-director deforms only in the axis of the prescribed macro displacement $\hat{u}_1$, as the micro-directors are already orientated parallel with that axis and thus the only micro-deformation activated is in $a_{\gamma 1}$. We recall there is only one micro-director whereby $a^0_{\gamma 1} = 1$, and include the only strain indices that change when deformed in this example ($r = s = j = 1$), as follows

$$2\,A_1\left(F_{11}a_{\gamma1}-\delta_{11}a^0_{\gamma1}\right)F_{11}=-A_2\left(a_{\gamma1}a_{\gamma1}-a^0_{\gamma1}a^0_{\gamma1}\right)a_{\gamma1} \tag{5.6}$$

$$2\,A_1\left(\lambda a_{\gamma1}-1\right)\lambda=-A_2\left(a_{\gamma1}a_{\gamma1}-1\right)a_{\gamma1}. \tag{5.7}$$

It is evident there exist two trivial micro-director deformation solutions to satisfy Eq. (5.7) for the following scenarios:

$$A_1\to\pm\infty \text{ or } A_2=0,\quad \text{then}\quad E^{(1)}_{\gamma1}\to 0, C^{(1)}_{\gamma1}\to 1,\quad \text{and thus}\quad a_{\gamma1}=1/\lambda \tag{5.8}$$

$$A_2\to\pm\infty \text{ or } A_1=0,\quad \text{then}\quad E^{(2)}_{\gamma1}\to 0, C^{(2)}_{\gamma1}\to 1,\quad \text{and thus}\quad a_{\gamma1}=1. \tag{5.9}$$

The solution to this homogeneous tension beam problem can be represented by rearranging Eq. (5.7) to achieve a cubic function in terms of the deformed micro-director length $f(a_{\gamma1})=0$ as follows

$$A_2a^3_{\gamma1}+a_{\gamma1}\left(2A_1\lambda^2-A_2\right)-2A_1\lambda=0. \tag{5.10}$$

A cubic function of the form $f(a_{\gamma1})=0$ can have a maximum of three solutions. In the context of this example, the solution achieved by the model will be the one that minimizes the energy in the system by way of the least micro-strain, and thus the closest solution to $a_{\gamma1}\to 1$. It can be seen in Figure 5.2a and Figure 5.2b, for varying $A_1$ and $A_2$ respectively, that non-trivial solutions are evident when $A_1\approx -A_2$, because it allows for larger mixed-scale strain and micro-scale strain whilst still maintaining the equilibrium in Eq. (5.7). The two trivial solutions of Eq. (5.8) and Eq. (5.9) are also clearly visible from the horizontal asymptotes. The model does not converge to a solution when the parameters are defined as $A_1=-A_2=A$, and substituting this special case into Eq. (5.10) gives

$$-Aa^3_{\gamma1}+2A\lambda^2a_{\gamma1}+Aa_{\gamma1}-2A\lambda=0 \tag{5.11}$$

$$-a^3_{\gamma1}+a_{\gamma1}\left(2\lambda^2+1\right)-2\lambda=0, \tag{5.12}$$

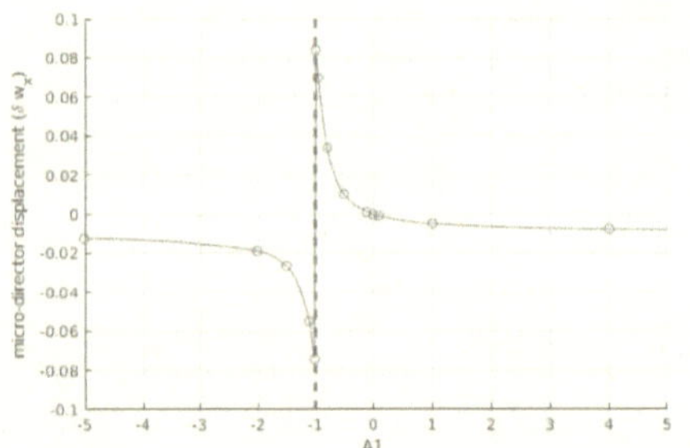


(a) Fixed $A_2=1$ kPa, varying $A_1$. Discontinuity at $A_2=-A_1=1$ kPa. Trivial solutions: y-intercept gives $a_1=1$ for $A_1=0$ kPa, and horizontal asymptote of $a_1\to 1/\lambda$ for $A_1\to\pm\infty$ kPa.

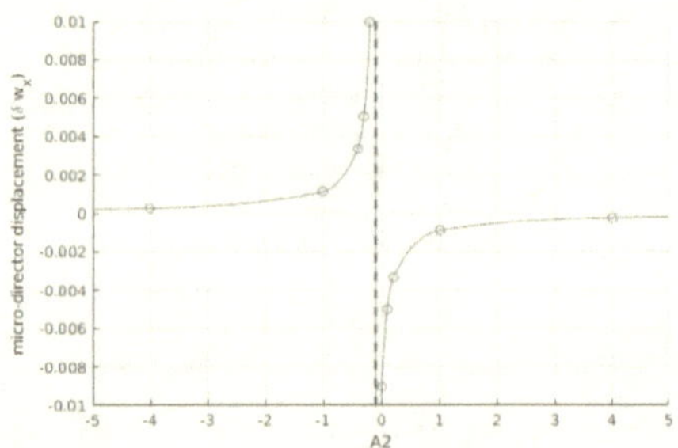


(b) Fixed $A_1=0.1$ kPa, varying $A_2$. Discontinuity at $A_1=-A_2=0.1$ kPa. Trivial solutions: y-intercept gives $a_1=1/\lambda$ for $A_2=0$ kPa, and horizontal asymptote of $a_1\to 1$ for $A_2\to\pm\infty$ kPa.

Fig. 5.2: Homogeneous deformation tension beam example: mixed-scale and micro-scale parameters influence on micro-director displacements for prescribed macro-stretch $\lambda=1.01$, and macro-scale linear isotropic material parameters $a_0=0.385$ kPa and $b_0=0.578$ kPa. Different fixed material parameters of $A_2=1$ kPa and $A_1=0.1$ kPa show that the discontinuity is independent of the material parameter magnitude, but it is dependent on the ratio of $A_1:A_2$.

and therefore the solution remains the same for any parameter $A$ provided $A_1 = -A_2$. For a prescribed macro-stretch $\lambda = 1.01$ the equation becomes

$$-a_{\gamma 1}^3 + 3.0402\, a_{\gamma 1} - 2.02 = 0, \tag{5.13}$$

and the graph of this function shown in Figure 5.3. The three solutions of the cubic function are

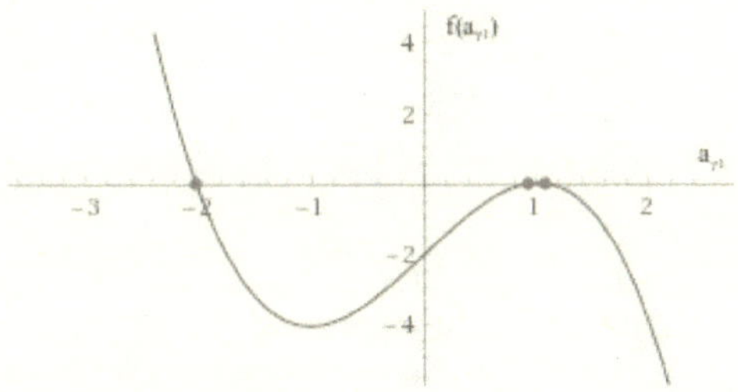


Fig. 5.3: Graph of the cubic function of Eq. (5.13), with $f(a_{\gamma 1})$ plotted on the y-axis and $a_{\gamma 1}$ plotted on the x-axis, for the homogeneous deformation tension beam problem with prescribed macro-stretch $\lambda = 1.01$, and micro-parameters $A_1 = -A_2$. The solutions of $f(a_{\gamma 1}) = 0$ for the possible deformed micro-director lengths are $a_{\gamma 1} = -2.01, 0.92, 1.09$, as labelled in red.

$a_{\gamma 1} = -2.01, 0.92, 1.09$, or in terms of micro-deformations $w_{\gamma 1} = -3.01, -0.08, 0.09$. The two solutions of $a_{\gamma 1} = 0.92, 1.09$ are almost equidistant from $a_{\gamma 1} = 1$, therefore it is difficult for the model to converge on a solution. A discontinuity in the solution is visible in both Figure 5.2a and Figure 5.2b when approaching $A_1 \to -A_2$, because approaching from one side of the discontinuity the solution of $a_{\gamma 1} < 1$ is closest to $a_{\gamma 1} = 1$ for $f(a_{\gamma 1}) = 0$, but from the other side of the discontinuity the solution of $a_{\gamma 1} > 1$ is closest to $a_{\gamma 1} = 1$ for $f(a_{\gamma 1}) = 0$. The understanding of the mixed-scale and micro-scale parameter relationships is necessary to ensure model solutions when using the micromorphic model. The same lack of a unique solution exists for a simple shear example when $A_1 = -A_2$ too; however, this is not examined in this study.

It is worth noting that it is possible to calculate the micro-director deformation of a homogeneous deformation tension beam problem without running the simulation but instead by simply finding the roots of Eq. (5.10), and selecting the root that is closest to $a_{\gamma 1} = 1$. Alternatively, if the desired micro-director deformation was known along with one of the micro-scale/mixed-scale parameters, it is possible to find the other corresponding calibrated micro-scale/mixed-scale parameter by substitution into Eq. (5.10), without the burden of calibrating from simulations using a calibration script.

### 5.1.2 Micro-director deformation and macro-traction vector contribution

The tension beam under homogeneous deformation discussed in Section 5.1.1 was very useful for understanding the fundamental deformation behaviour of the micro-director, and hence the same example is further explored here. In addition to the lack of a unique solution uncovered, it was observed that the micro-director does not necessarily stretch when the bulk material is stretched, nor does it necessarily contract when the bulk material is compressed. It was previously displayed in Figure 5.2 that for prescribed axial stretching of the macro-scale (bulk material) the micro-director could either stretch or contract depending upon the mixed-scale material parameter $A_1$ in relation to the micro-scale material parameter $A_2$. Not only does this have an effect on the deformation of the micro-director, but it also affects the external macro-traction vector $\hat{\mathbf{t}}^{(\mathbf{n})}$ of Eq. (4.57) through $\mathbf{S}^{(1)}$, and therefore the significance of $\hat{\mathbf{t}}^{(\mathbf{n})}$ will now be explained.

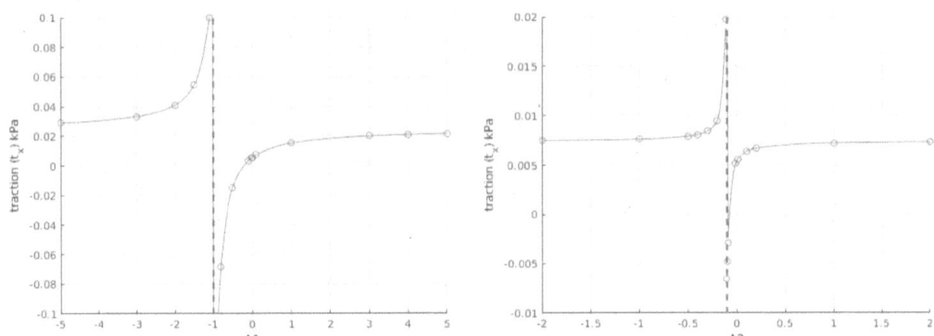


(a) Fixed $A_2 = 1$ kPa, varying $A_1$. Discontinuity at $A_2 = -A_1 = 1$ kPa.

(b) Fixed $A_1 = 0.1$ kPa, varying $A_2$. Discontinuity at $A_1 = -A_2 = 0.1$ kPa.

Fig. 5.4: Homogeneous deformation tension beam example: mixed-scale/micro-scale parameter influence on macro-scale traction vector $\hat{\mathbf{t}}^{(\mathbf{n})}$ for prescribed macro-stretch $\lambda = 1.01$, and macro-scale linear isotropic material parameters $a_0 = 0.385$ kPa and $b_0 = 0.578$ kPa.

The resulting macro-traction vector $\hat{\mathbf{t}}^{(\mathbf{n})}$ depending on the ratio $A_1 : A_2$ for prescribed macro-stretch $\lambda = 1.01$, and constant macro-scale linear isotropic material parameters $a_0 = 0.385$ kPa and $b_0 = 0.578$ kPa of Eq. (4.66), can be seen in Figure 5.4a and Figure 5.4b. For a typical classical model, we find that increasing a material stiffness parameter will increase the overall stiffness of the material, i.e. for a displacement-driven problem the resulting components of $\hat{\mathbf{t}}^{(\mathbf{n})}$ should increase when a material parameter is increased. However, we see in Figure 5.4a that this is not always the case for the micromorphic model, because $\hat{t}_1^{(\mathbf{n})}$ can also decrease when increasing $A_1$. For example, from $A_1 = -1.1\,\mathrm{kPa}$ to $A_1 = -0.1\,\mathrm{kPa}$, we find $\hat{t}_1^{(\mathbf{n})}$ decreases, despite an increase in $A_1$. This phenomenon is even more complex when both $A_1$ and $A_2$ are increased. For a physical system, if two materials with identical geometry are deformed in the same way, the material that requires the largest components of $\hat{\mathbf{t}}^{(\mathbf{n})}$ to deform is the stiffer of the two materials. Again, for a typical classical model this is achieved by increasing the material parameter. However, for the micromorphic model we find that increasing a mixed-scale or micro-scale material parameter does not necessarily increase $\hat{t}_1^{(\mathbf{n})}$, and therefore it is best to use the resulting components of $\hat{\mathbf{t}}^{(\mathbf{n})}$ for a displacement-driven problem as a proxy for the overall material stiffness, rather than interpreting that directly from the material parameters.

The explanation of the deformation of the micro-director and its subsequent effect on the macro-scale traction vector $\hat{\mathbf{t}}^{(\mathbf{n})}$ is attributed to the equilibrium equation over the micro-scale degrees of freedom that was reduced to the clear representation of Eq. (5.3) from Section 5.1.1. We can approximate Eq. (5.3), knowing that for small strains we find that $F_{11} \approx a_{\gamma 1} \approx 1$, for one micro-director $\gamma = 1$, and absorbing the factor 2 into $A_1$ given that the factor is dependent on the chosen handling of the mixed-scale basis vector double contraction mentioned in Section 4.3.1, with

$$A_1 E^{(1)\gamma 1} \approx -A_2 E^{(2)\gamma\gamma} \tag{5.14}$$

$$S^{(1)\gamma 1} \approx -S^{(2)\gamma\gamma}. \tag{5.15}$$

It is clear that the mixed-scale stress and the micro-scale stress have to be approximately equal and opposite to enforce the equilibrium over the micro-scale degrees of freedom. This is the case for any combination of $A_1 : A_2$ since $E^{(1)\gamma 1}$ and $E^{(2)\gamma\gamma}$ will adjust accordingly to maintain the equilibrium. This means that if both material parameters $A_1$ and $A_2$ are positive, then one of the strains must be positive and the other negative to enforce Eq. (5.14). In the case of the tension beam this means that the micro-director must contract $w_{\gamma 1} < 0$ under macro-scale prescribed stretch $u_1 > 0$ and $A_1, A_2 > 0$, as this enables $E^{(1)\gamma 1} > 0$ and $E^{(2)\gamma\gamma} < 0$, and thus Eq. (5.14) is satisfied. We note that the mixed-scale strain $E^{(1)\gamma 1}$ can still be positive when the micro-director shrinks provided the macro-stretch outweighs the shrinking of the micro-director ($F_{11} > 1/a_{\gamma 1}$), as follows

$$E^{(1)\gamma 1} > 0, \quad \text{if} \quad w_{\gamma 1} < 0, \quad \because \quad C^{(1)\gamma 1} = F_{s1} a_{\gamma s} > 1, \quad \text{if} \quad F_{11} > 1/a_{\gamma 1}. \tag{5.16}$$

In terms of what is anticipated in reality from a fibrous material subjected to prescribed stretching of the bulk material, a complimentary stretch of the fibre would be expected. However, it has just been shown that this would not seem possible using positive mixed-scale and micro-scale material parameters. This artifact of Sansour's micromorphic model will be discussed further in Section 5.3.

In Section 5.1.1 the trivial solutions of $E^{(1)\gamma 1} \to 0$ in Eq. (5.8) and $E^{(2)\gamma\gamma} \to 0$ in Eq. (5.9) were explained in relation to enforcing the equilibrium. However, in zones of $A_1 \sim -A_2$, we find that the LHS and RHS of Eq. (5.14) can both now be large whilst still equal. There is no trivial solution when $A_1 \sim -A_2$ because $F_{11} \neq 1$ for prescribed macro-stretch, therefore zero micro-director deformation would result in $E^{(1)\gamma 1} > 0$ and $E^{(2)\gamma\gamma} = 0$, therefore the equilibrium would fail. The term $A_1 E^{(1)\gamma 1}$ or rather $S^{(1)\gamma 1}$ features in the macro-equilibrium of Eq. (4.57) and thus contributes to the macro-scale traction vector $\hat{\mathbf{t}}^{(\mathbf{n})}(\mathbf{S}^{(0)}, \mathbf{S}^{(1)})$. The stretch or contraction of the micro-director dictates the sign of $E^{(1)\gamma 1}$, so that when multiplied with $A_1$ the mixed-scale stress $S^{(1)\gamma 1}$ will be either positive or negative and therefore increase or decrease $\hat{t}_1^{(\mathbf{n})}$. Using the example of Eq. (5.8) to illustrate an increase or decrease $\hat{t}_1^{(\mathbf{n})}$, we define $A_1 \to \infty$, and hence know that $E^{(1)\gamma 1} \to 0$ to satisfy the equilibrium, or $C^{(1)\gamma 1} \to 1$ and thus $a_{\gamma 1} \to 1/F_{11}$. This means that $w_{\gamma 1} < 0$, and thus $E^{(2)\gamma\gamma} < 0$. Therefore, whether a positive or negative contribution is made to $\hat{t}_1^{(\mathbf{n})}$ through Eq. (4.57) depends on the sign of the undefined parameter $A_2$, as to whether $E^{(1)\gamma 1} \to 0^+$, or $E^{(1)\gamma 1} \to 0^-$, as follows

$$\underbrace{A_1}_{\to\infty} \times \underbrace{E^{(1)\gamma 1}}_{\to 0^+} + \underbrace{A_2}_{+ve} \times \underbrace{E^{(2)\gamma\gamma}}_{-ve} = 0, \qquad \therefore \quad \left(E^{(1)\gamma 1} > 0,\, S^{(1)\gamma 1} > 0,\, \hat{t}_1^{(\mathbf{n})} \uparrow\right) \tag{5.17}$$

$$\underbrace{A_1}_{\to\infty} \times \underbrace{E^{(1)\gamma 1}}_{\to 0^-} + \underbrace{A_2}_{-ve} \times \underbrace{E^{(2)\gamma\gamma}}_{-ve} = 0, \qquad \therefore \quad \left(E^{(1)\gamma 1} < 0,\, S^{(1)\gamma 1} < 0,\, \hat{t}_1^{(\mathbf{n})} \downarrow\right). \tag{5.18}$$

We find for Eq. (5.17) that $S^{(1)\gamma 1} > 0$ and thus $\hat{t}_1^{(\mathbf{n})}$ is increased through Eq. (4.57), whereas in Eq. (5.18) we find $S^{(1)\gamma 1} < 0$ and thus $\hat{t}_1^{(\mathbf{n})}$ is decreased through Eq. (4.57), where the only difference is the sign of $A_2$. In order to understand the effect of the material parameter ratio $A_1 : A_2$ on the overall material stiffness using $\hat{\mathbf{t}}^{(\mathbf{n})}$ as a proxy, a range of mixed-scale and micro-scale material parameter ratios were simulated. The behaviour of the micro-director and the overall material stiffness response (using the resulting macro-traction vector $\hat{\mathbf{t}}^{(\mathbf{n})}$ as a proxy for this) is tabulated in Table 5.1, and the effect of making either of the material parameters very large is seen in Table 5.2.

Table 5.1: Table of material parameter ratio $A_1 : A_2$ effect on the overall material stiffness, using the resulting macro-traction vector $\hat{\mathbf{t}}^{(\mathbf{n})}$ as a proxy for this, for prescribed macro-scale displacement.

| $A_1$ | $A_2$ | Relative | $w_1$ | $E^{(1)\gamma 1}$ | $S^{(1)\gamma 1}$ | Material stiffness (proxy - $\hat{t}_1^{(\mathbf{n})}$) |
|---|---|---|---|---|---|---|
| $A_1 > 0$ | $A_2 > 0$ | - | -ve: $1/F_{11} < a_{\gamma 1} < 1$ | +ve | $A_1 \times E^{(1)\gamma 1} = (+) \text{ x } (+) = +\text{ve}$ | Stiffer |
| $A_1 > 0$ | $A_2 = 0$ | $\lvert A_1 \rvert > \lvert A_2 \rvert$ | -ve: $a_{\gamma 1} = 1/F_{11}$ | 0 | $A_1 \times E^{(1)\gamma 1} = (+) \text{ x } (0) = 0$ | no contribution |
| $A_1 > 0$ | $A_2 < 0$ | $\lvert A_1 \rvert > \lvert A_2 \rvert$ | -ve: $a_{\gamma 1} < 1/F_{11}$ | -ve | $A_1 \times E^{(1)\gamma 1} = (+) \text{ x } (-) = -\text{ve}$ | Weaker |
| $A_1 > 0$ | $A_2 < 0$ | $\lvert A_1 \rvert < \lvert A_2 \rvert$ | +ve: $a_{\gamma 1} > 1$ | +ve | $A_1 \times E^{(1)\gamma 1} = (+) \text{ x } (+) = +\text{ve}$ | Stiffer |
| $A_1 < 0$ | $A_2 > 0$ | $\lvert A_1 \rvert > \lvert A_2 \rvert$ | -ve: $a_{\gamma 1} < 1/F_{11}$ | -ve | $A_1 \times E^{(1)\gamma 1} = (-) \text{ x } (-) = +\text{ve}$ | Stiffer |
| $A_1 < 0$ | $A_2 > 0$ | $\lvert A_1 \rvert < \lvert A_2 \rvert$ | +ve: $a_{\gamma 1} > 1$ | +ve | $A_1 \times E^{(1)\gamma 1} = (-) \text{ x } (+) = -\text{ve}$ | Weaker |
| $A_1 < 0$ | $A_2 = 0$ | $\lvert A_1 \rvert > \lvert A_2 \rvert$ | -ve: $a_{\gamma 1} = 1/F_{11}$ | 0 | $A_1 \times E^{(1)\gamma 1} = (-) \text{ x } (0) = 0$ | no contribution |
| $A_1 < 0$ | $A_2 < 0$ | - | -ve: $1/F_{11} < a_{\gamma 1} < 1$ | +ve | $A_1 \times E^{(1)\gamma 1} = (-) \text{ x } (+) = -\text{ve}$ | Weaker |

Table 5.2: Table of large material parameter values effect on the overall material stiffness, using the resulting macro-traction vector $\hat{\mathbf{t}}^{(\mathbf{n})}$ as a proxy for this, for prescribed macro-scale displacement.

| $A_1$ | $A_2$ | $E^{(1)\gamma 1}$ | $w_{\gamma 1}$ | $E^{(2)\gamma\gamma}$ | Equilibrium | Material stiffness (proxy - $\hat{t}_1^{(\mathbf{n})}$) |
|---|---|---|---|---|---|---|
| $A_1 \to \infty$ | $A_2 > 0$ | $0^+$ | -ve: $a_{\gamma 1} \to 1/F_{11}$ | -ve | $A_1 \times E^{(1)\gamma 1} + A_2 \times E^{(2)\gamma\gamma} = 0$<br>$\infty \times 0^+ + (+) \times (-) = 0$ | Stiffer |
| $A_1 \to \infty$ | $A_2 < 0$ | $0^-$ | -ve: $a_{\gamma 1} \to 1/F_{11}$ | -ve | $A_1 \times E^{(1)\gamma 1} + A_2 \times E^{(2)\gamma\gamma} = 0$<br>$\infty \times 0^- + (-) \times (-) = 0$ | Softer |
| $A_1 > 0$ | $A_2 \to \infty$ | +ve | -ve: $a_{\gamma 1} \to 1^-$ | $0^-$ | $A_1 \times E^{(1)\gamma 1} + A_2 \times E^{(2)\gamma\gamma} = 0$<br>$(+) \times (+) + \infty \times 0^- = 0$ | Stiffer |
| $A_1 < 0$ | $A_2 \to \infty$ | +ve | -ve: $a_{\gamma 1} \to 1^+$ | $0^+$ | $A_1 \times E^{(1)\gamma 1} + A_2 \times E^{(2)\gamma\gamma} = 0$<br>$(-) \times (+) + \infty \times 0^+ = 0$ | Softer |

The interdependence of $A_1 : A_2$ is evidently crucial. Unlike classical models where a large material parameter results in a stiffer material, that is not necessarily the case for the micromorphic model as manipulating the ratio of $A_1 : A_2$ can have a greater impact on the material stiffness (quantified using $\mathbf{t}^{(\mathbf{n})}$ as a proxy) than simply making $A_1$ very large on its own, or $A_2$, as seen in Figure 5.4a and Figure 5.4b. Furthermore, cautious selection of material parameters is necessary, because it is visible in Figure 5.4a and Figure 5.4b that it is possible to get a compressive macro-traction vector $\hat{\mathbf{t}}^{(\mathbf{n})}$ for prescribed axial stretching, which is clearly a non-physical result.

## 5.2 Artifacts of displacement based strain

It was shown in Section 5.1.2 that for positive mixed-scale and positive micro-scale material parameters, the micro-director seemingly has no option but to contract even though a stretch has been prescribed in $\mathbf{u}$ because of the equilibrium over the micro-scale degrees of freedom $A_1\mathbf{E}^{(1)} \approx -A_2\mathbf{E}^{(2)}$. This artifact of the micromorphic model does not match what is expected of a fibrous material under axial stretching in reality, as the fibres in turn would also be expected to stretch. For instance, the grain in wood will also stretch when the wood is stretched, similarly the steel in reinforced concrete will stretch if the concrete is stretched. The use of all positive material parameters would seem the only physically justifiable option because the strain energy of all the scales should be positive. This means that for the macro-scale the bulk material will store energy when deformed, for the mixed-scale the cohesion or friction between the bulk material and fibres will store energy when deformed, and finally for the micro-scale the fibres themselves will store energy when deformed. Furthermore, positive material parameters ensure convexity of the strain energy function [36, 92]. Consequently, in the case of axial stretching, it would be desirable that all three scales (macro/mixed/micro) produce strain and stress that is representative of tension, such that the components of $S^{(0)kl}, S^{(1)j\gamma}, S^{(2)\lambda\mu} > 0$ in the direction of the prescribed stretch $\bar{u}_i$.

For the same homogeneous deformation tension beam example of Section 5.1 with the same linear constitutive law, it was hoped that by applying a tensile *Neumann* boundary micro-traction $\hat{\mathbf{q}}_\gamma^{(\mathbf{n})}$ or a stretching *Dirichlet* boundary micro-deformation $\bar{\mathbf{w}}_\gamma$ on the micro-director degrees of freedom, it would force the micro-directors to stretch. Unfortunately, this was not found to be the case from the results of this study. For a purely force-driven model on both macro-scale and micro-scale degrees of freedom, with a tensile boundary macro-traction $\hat{t}_1^{(\mathbf{n})} = 0.01\,\text{kPa}$ and tensile micro-traction $\hat{q}_{\gamma 1}^{(\mathbf{n})} = 0.01\,\text{kPa}$ both on the member's free end, and with prescribed zero boundary macro-displacement $\bar{\mathbf{u}} = \mathbf{0}$ and zero boundary micro-deformation $\bar{\mathbf{w}}_\gamma = \mathbf{0}$ on the member's fixed end, we still end up with the micro-director contracting through the majority of the member, as seen in Figure 5.5a. Similarly, for a purely displacement-driven model on both macro-scale and micro-scale degrees of freedom, with a prescribed stretch boundary macro-displacement $\bar{u}_1 = 0.1\,\text{m}$ and stretch boundary micro-deformation $\bar{w}_{\gamma 1} = 0.1$ on the non-zero *Dirichlet* boundary, and with prescribed zero boundary macro-displacement $\bar{\mathbf{u}} = \mathbf{0}$ and zero boundary micro-deformation $\bar{\mathbf{w}}_\gamma = \mathbf{0}$ on the member's fixed end, we also end up with micro-director contracting through the majority of the member, as seen in Figure 5.5b. Clearly, both of these results seem to be non-physical artifacts of the model. This artifact of micro-directors contracting under bulk material tension is also visible in the micromorphic example in Figure 6(b)-(e) of von Hoegen et al. (2017), which serves as independent verification, although the issue was not highlighted nor discussed there.

The author has established a novel explanation for this artifact of the model, and will now document it here. In order to understand why Sansour's version of the micromorphic model behaves this way, we start from the variational formulation of Eq. (4.53), and shall ignore higher-order terms ($l_\alpha \ll 1$), as was done in this study. If we were to take a perpendicular cut $\partial\mathcal{B}_x$ through the tension beam's length (x-axis) at any point, and after applying *Gauss*' divergence theorem to Eq. (4.53) to produce a surface integral representing the internal force acting normal to $\partial\mathcal{B}_x$, in the absence of body forces, and with the external traction $\hat{t}_r^{(\mathbf{n})}$ on the opposite end that keeps the divided member in equilibrium, we arrive at the following energy balance over macro-scale degrees of freedom

(a) Micro-director deformations $w_{\gamma 1}$ for tensile boundary macro-traction $\hat{t}_1^{(\mathbf{n})} = 0.01\,\text{kPa}$, and tensile boundary micro-traction $\hat{q}_{\gamma 1}^{(\mathbf{n})} = 0.01\,\text{kPa}$ on free end (right face).

(b) Micro-director deformations $w_{\gamma 1}$ for boundary macro-displacement $\bar{u}_1 = 0.1\,\text{m}$, and micro-boundary displacement $\bar{w}_{\gamma 1} = 0.1$ on the non-zero *Dirichlet* boundary (right face).

Fig. 5.5: Homogeneous deformation tension beam example: boundary micro-conditions influence on micro-director deformations. Macro-scale linear isotropic material parameters $a_0 = 0.385$ kPa and $b_0 = 0.578$ kPa in Eq. (4.66), and $A_1 = A_2 = 1$ kPa in Eq. (4.73). Prescribed zero boundary macro-displacement $\bar{\mathbf{u}} = \mathbf{0}$ and zero boundary micro-deformation $\bar{\mathbf{w}}_\alpha = \mathbf{0}$ on fixed end (left face). Despite tensile boundary micro-traction or stretching boundary micro-deformation at the displacing end of the beam, the micro-director still contracts in the majority of the member.

$$\int_{\partial \mathcal{B}_x} [S^{(0)kl} F_{rk} + S^{(1)l\gamma} a_{\gamma r}] n_l \delta u_r \, dA - \int_{\partial \mathcal{B}_\mathcal{N}} \hat{t}_r^{(\mathbf{n})} \delta u_r \, dA = 0 \, . \tag{5.19}$$

Furthermore, since the problem is defined to produce homogeneous deformation, the surface area $A$ of $\partial \mathcal{B}_x$ is the same no matter where the cut along the x-axis is taken, because the cross-section dimensions are the same everywhere. Thus we arrive at

$$\int_{\delta \mathcal{B}} \left( S^{(0)kl} F_{rk} n_l + S^{(1)l\gamma} a_{\gamma r} n_l - \hat{t}_r^{(\mathbf{n})} \right) \delta u_r \, dA = 0 \, , \tag{5.20}$$

and since $\delta \mathbf{u}$ is a free variation, we find that at any perpendicular cross-section $\partial \mathcal{B}_x$ in the member

$$S^{(0)kl} F_{rk} n_l + S^{(1)l\gamma} a_{\gamma r} n_l = \hat{t}_r^{(\mathbf{n})} \qquad \text{(Homogenous deformation)}, \tag{5.21}$$

and therefore at any point along the beam the surface integral is satisfied and gives $\mathbf{S}^{(0)}, \mathbf{S}^{(1)} \propto \hat{\mathbf{t}}^{(\mathbf{n})}$ in the direction of the surface normal at $\partial \mathcal{B}_x$. We can see this is satisfied by plotting the stresses at *Gauss* points along the beams length, as seen in Figure 5.6, whereby $S^{(0)11} + S^{(1)\gamma 1} = 0.015 - 0.005 = \hat{t}_1^{(\mathbf{n})}$ at all points in the beam.

However, we cannot reach the same conclusion for the energy balance over the micro-scale degrees of freedom. Instead, the variational formulation of Eq. (4.53), again ignoring higher-order terms ($l_\alpha \ll 1$) and with no body forces, contains terms in the volume integral that have a variant in the form of a displacement $\delta a_{\gamma r}$ - instead of a strain gradient $\delta a_{\gamma r,l}$ - as follows

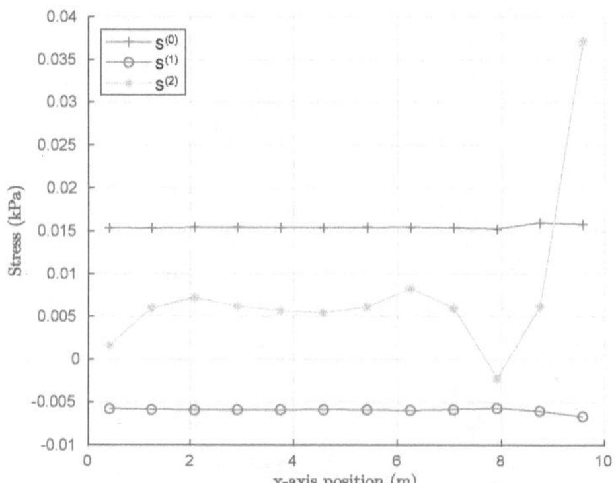


Fig. 5.6: Homogeneous deformation tension beam example: Graph of stresses at *Gauss* points along beam's axis for tensile boundary macro-traction $\hat{t}_1^{(\mathbf{n})} = 0.01\,\text{kPa}$, and tensile boundary micro-traction $\hat{q}_{\gamma 1}^{(\mathbf{n})} = 0.01\,\text{kPa}$ on free end (right face). We note that $S^{(0)11} + S^{(1)\gamma 1} = 0.015 - 0.005 = \hat{t}_1^{(\mathbf{n})}$ at all points in the beam.

$$\int_{\mathcal{B}} [S^{(1)J\gamma} F_{rj} + S^{(2)\gamma\mu} a_{\mu r}] \delta a_{\gamma r}\, dV - \int_{\delta\mathcal{B}_{\mathcal{N}}} \hat{q}_{\gamma r}^{(\mathbf{n})} \delta a_{\gamma r}\, dA = 0. \tag{5.22}$$

This is a crucial difference because it means that *Gauss*' divergence theorem cannot be used to transform the volume integral into a surface integral at any cross-section $\partial\mathcal{B}_x$ as we did previously to arrive at Eq. (5.19). As such, over the micro-scale degrees of freedom, we find only the volume integral must be satisfied, but the surface integral at any point along the beam $\partial\mathcal{B}_x$ is no longer required and therefore at any point on a homogeneous tension beam $\mathbf{S}^{(1)}$, $\mathbf{S}^{(2)} \not\propto \hat{\mathbf{q}}_\gamma^{(\mathbf{n})}$ in the direction of the surface normal at $\partial\mathcal{B}_x$, as seen in Figure 5.6. This allows for spurious, non-physical micro-director deformations that were evident in Figure 5.5a and Figure 5.5b. We can see the micro-director deformations during prescribed macro-boundary stretch $\lambda = 1.01$ for a range of boundary micro-tractions $\hat{q}_{\gamma 1}^{(\mathbf{n})}$ in Figure 5.7a and micro-director deformation relative to the end node in Figure 5.7b. The erratic nature of the micro-director deformation solution is clearly visible in Figure 5.7a, although the relative behaviour follows a pattern to some extent in Figure 5.7b. This behaviour should be investigated further in future work.

We also notice from Figure 5.7a that the director displacement can fluctuate from positive and negative at one node to the next. This brings into question a major concern the author has with Sansour's version of the micromorphic model. The model is based on the concept of a macro-derivative and a micro-derivative, which together make up the generalized deformation-gradient of Eq. (4.24). However, the micro-derivative is taken analytically $\partial(\zeta^\alpha \mathbf{a}_\alpha)/\partial\zeta^\gamma = \mathbf{a}_\gamma$, instead of using gradient shape functions as it typically done in classical mechanics with $\mathbf{u}_{,i}$. This results in dominant micromorphic mixed-scale and micro-scale strain measures based on the deformation measure $\mathbf{a}_\gamma$ as a proxy for strain, and not strain gradient fields $\mathbf{a}_{\gamma,i}$.

The author believes that using displacement as a strain measure rather than a strain gradient allows for non-physical model solutions, because the volume integral in Eq. (5.22) can still be satisfied by

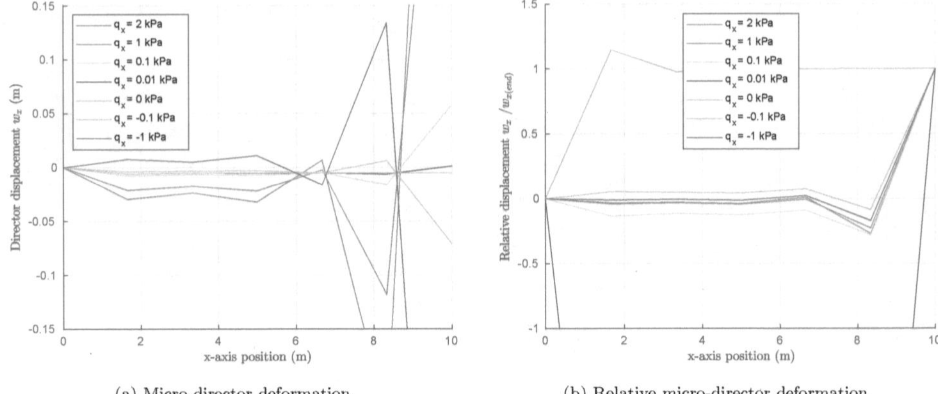


(a) Micro-director deformation.

(b) Relative micro-director deformation.

Fig. 5.7: Homogeneous deformation tension beam example: boundary micro-traction $\hat{\mathbf{q}}^{(\mathbf{n})}$ influence on micro-director deformation along beam length for prescribed macro-stretch $\lambda = 1.01$, and macro-scale linear isotropic material parameters $a_0 = 0.385$ kPa and $b_0 = 0.578$ kPa, and material parameters $A_1 = A_2 = 1$ kPa.

non-physical displacements $\mathbf{w}_\gamma$ at any node, without affecting the strain gradient of adjacent nodes, as the formulation is not reliant on $\mathbf{a}_{\gamma,i}$. In other words, for strain gradient displacement solutions, the strain gradient is affected by strains at adjacent nodes, and thus a more realistic gradient is achieved. However, this is not enforced for the displacement strain measure, and hence we saw in Figure 5.7a the micro-director displacement could jump from positive to negative from one node to the next. Additionally, the author also cautions the use of an analytical geometry in a finite element approximation problem.

The use of mixed-scale and micro-scale strain measures based upon deformation and not strain gradients can be challenged succinctly using the following counter-hypothesis: "Does it make sense that in a tension beam, if the micro-director is fixed at one end and stretched at the other end, the stress in the micro-director at the fixed end is zero?". To elaborate, if a fibrous material is fixed at one end by both the bulk material and its fibres, and then both the bulk material and the fibres are stretched by a prescribed amount at the other end, the fibre would be under stress along its entire length including at the end at which it is fixed. However, for Sansour's micromorphic model, the micro-director strain measure is calculated directly from micro-director deformation, and since the micro-director deformation was fixed at this point $\bar{a}_{\gamma 1} = 1$, we find $C^{(2)\gamma\gamma} = \bar{a}_{\gamma 1}\bar{a}_{\gamma 1} = 1$, and thus the *Green* strain $E^{(2)\gamma\gamma} = 0$ at the fixed node. The micro-director stress is therefore $S^{(2)\gamma\gamma} = 0$, and this does not seem physically representative given the scenario. Furthermore, we can extend this scenario for a beam of 1 m length and another beam of 10 m length. If the prescribed non-zero boundary micro-deformation is $\bar{w}_{\gamma 1} = 0.1$, then the micro-stress $S^{(2)\gamma\gamma}$ is the same for both beams at the boundaries. However, if the strain were gradient based then the micro-stress $S^{(2)\gamma\gamma}$ would be much larger in the shorter beam, as the strain gradient is much larger for the same displacement over a shorter length $\partial w_{\gamma 1}/\partial L_1 > \partial w_{\gamma 1}/\partial L_{10}$.

The issue perhaps hinges on what the micro-directors represent physically in the material: are they continuous throughout the body, connected at every point, or do they stand alone in the body and are not interconnected? In the former case of continuous fibres, one envisages reinforced concrete, where the steel is continuously connected throughout the concrete body. In the latter case of discontinuous fibres, we consider a fibre-reinforced concrete, whereby the concrete contains short discrete fibres, such as synthetic fibres. These small fibres help change the properties of the bulk material, but are not joined together along the bulk material. In explanation of the findings, the author hypothesises that Sansour's deformation based micromorphic approach is best suited for discrete fibrous materials where the fibres are not continuous through the body.

*Mathematical explanation for micro-director contracting*

It was proposed by the author that deformation based strain measures allow for non-physical micro-director displacements, as shown in the tension beam example with contracting micro-directors. A mathematical explanation to support why the micro-directors in the tension beam contract for a prescribed boundary macro-stretching and positive material parameters $A_1, A_2 > 0$, as seen in Figure 5.5a and Figure 5.5b, was developed by the author. The explanation does not serve as a definitive explanation based upon the fundamental theory, but rather addresses all the parameters that populate the finite element equation system to identify what might be causing the micro-directors to shrink unexpectedly.

The explanation will be simplified as much as possible by using a one element simulation for the same tension beam example of Figure 5.1, because the same justification would apply for any additional elements. Also, we will not prescribe boundary conditions on the micro-director to further simplify the example. In the case of the tension beam example with only one hexahedral element of 8 nodes, which has 4 fixed nodes at one end $\bar{u}_{E(x)} = 0$, and prescribed macro-boundary displacement $\bar{u}_{E(x)} = 0.1$ for the remaining 4 nodes on the other end of the element, we find that all the nodes in the system are essential or *Dirichlet* conditions for the macro-scale degrees of freedom $\mathbf{u}_E$. Therefore, the only free degrees of freedom to solve for the model are the micro-scale degrees of freedom in $\mathbf{a}_F$. We now remind ourselves of the partitioning of a FEM system:

$$\begin{bmatrix} \mathbf{R}_E \\ \mathbf{0} \end{bmatrix} = \underbrace{\begin{bmatrix} \mathbf{K}_{EE} & \mathbf{K}_{EF} \\ \mathbf{K}_{FE} & \mathbf{K}_{FF} \end{bmatrix} \begin{bmatrix} \mathbf{d}_E \\ \mathbf{d}_F \end{bmatrix}}_{\text{(Internal Force)}} - \underbrace{\begin{bmatrix} \mathbf{F}_E \\ \mathbf{F}_F \end{bmatrix}}_{\text{(External Force)}} . \tag{5.23}$$

We solve the free nodal displacements using the bottom row equilibrium (partition) of Eq. (5.23), and since in the case of a displacement-driven model without body forces, there is no external force applied to free nodes $\mathbf{F}_F = \mathbf{0}$, we find

$$\mathbf{K}_{FF}\mathbf{d}_F = -\mathbf{K}_{FE}\mathbf{d}_E. \tag{5.24}$$

For the beam under axial stretch in the x-axis direction, we substitute the only relevant terms for free nodal displacements $\mathbf{d}_{F(a_1)}$, because it was found in the simulation that $\mathbf{d}_{F(a_2)}, \mathbf{d}_{F(a_3)} \approx 0$ since they are orthogonal to the loading direction, and non-zero prescribed displacements $\mathbf{d}_{E(u_1)}$ as follows

$$\mathbf{K}_{FF(a_1)}\mathbf{d}_{F(a_1)} = -\mathbf{K}_{FE(u_1)}\mathbf{d}_{E(u_1)}. \tag{5.25}$$

Furthermore, we know that any row of our partitioned system in Eq. (5.25) must be in equilibrium, and thus we can simply examine a single row. For example, if we look at an arbitrary node that we shall call $\Theta$ and isolate its micro-scale degree of freedom $(a_1)$, this will correspond to a single row in Eq. (5.25) such that

$$\mathbf{K}_{\Theta(a_1),F(a_1)} \cdot \mathbf{d}_{F(a_1)} = -\mathbf{K}_{\Theta(a_1),E(u_1)} \cdot \mathbf{d}_{E(u_1)}. \tag{5.26}$$

In the case where all the material parameters are positive, we find that every entry of the various stress derivatives is positive $\mathbb{H}^{(i)} = \partial S^{(i)}/\partial C^{(i)} \geq 0$, and we can substitute the dominant linearized terms from Eq. (A.27) of Appendix A.2.1 into the stiffness tangent terms of $\mathbf{K}_{\Theta(a_1)|F(a_1)}$ and $\mathbf{K}_{\Theta(a_1)|E(u_1)}$. Additionally, the variant $\delta\mathbf{a}$ in both $\mathbf{K}_{\Theta(a_1)|F(a_1)}$ and $\mathbf{K}_{\Theta(a_1)|E(u_1)}$ is approximated from *Gauss* (quadrature) points with shape functions $(N_i)$ which are always positive, such that $\delta\mathbf{a} \rightarrow N_i > 0$. The remaining variant $\delta\mathbf{u}_{,i}$ in $\mathbf{K}_{\Theta(a_1)|E(u_1)}$ is approximated from gauss points using derivative shape functions $(B_{r,i})$, and for this simulation the non-zero essential nodes sit on the maximum x-axis value face, and thus $\delta u_{1,1} \rightarrow B_{1,1} > 0$. Finally, for small strain we know $F_{11}, a_1 \approx 1$. Substituting the aforementioned and considering relevant indices, we find for the row of node $\Theta(a_1)$ of the partitioned system:

$$\begin{bmatrix} \underbrace{\mathbb{H}^{(1)1\gamma1\lambda}}_{(+ve)} \underbrace{F_{11}}_{1} \underbrace{F_{11}}_{1} \underbrace{\underbrace{\Delta a_{\lambda1}}_{(\text{node } \Theta)}}_{(+ve)} \underbrace{\underbrace{\delta a_{\gamma1}}_{(\text{free nodes})}}_{(+ve)} \\ + \\ 4\,\underbrace{\mathbb{H}^{(2)\tau\omega\eta\phi}}_{(+ve)} \underbrace{a_{\phi1}}_{1} \underbrace{a_{\omega1}}_{1} \underbrace{\underbrace{\Delta a_{\eta1}}_{(\text{node } \Theta)}}_{(+ve)} \underbrace{\underbrace{\delta a_{\tau1}}_{(\text{free nodes})}}_{(+ve)} \end{bmatrix} \cdot \left[\mathbf{d}_{F(a_1)}\right] = - \begin{bmatrix} \underbrace{\mathbb{H}^{(1)1\gamma1\lambda}}_{(+ve)} \underbrace{a_{\lambda1}}_{1} \underbrace{F_{11}}_{1} \underbrace{\underbrace{\Delta a_{\gamma1}}_{(\text{node } \Theta)}}_{(+ve)} \underbrace{\underbrace{\delta u_{1,1}}_{(\text{Ess. nodes})}}_{(+ve)} \end{bmatrix} \cdot \left[\underbrace{\mathbf{d}_{E(u_1)}}_{(+ve)}\right], \tag{5.27}$$

which can be simplified for the purpose of this exercise to the indicative form

$$\underbrace{\mathbf{K}_{\Theta(a_1),F(a_1)}}_{(+ve)} \cdot \mathbf{d}_{F(a_1)} = -\underbrace{\mathbf{K}_{\Theta(a_1),E(u_1)}}_{(+ve)} \cdot \underbrace{\mathbf{d}_{E(u_1)}}_{(+ve)}. \tag{5.28}$$

Clearly, in order for Eq. (5.28) to be satisfied the majority of free nodes must solve to have negative micro-director displacements

$$\therefore \mathbf{d}_{F(a_1)} \overset{!}{=} -ve, \tag{5.29}$$

and thus the directors must contract, which compliments what was seen in Figure 5.5a and Figure 5.5b. It is useful now to compare the equation system of Eq. (5.25) to that of a classical example, in order to understand what drives the classical degrees of freedom $\delta\mathbf{d}_{F(\mathbf{u})}$ of free nodes to stretch under tension. For a classical model of the same tension beam example, but with two or more elements otherwise there would be no free nodes to solve, we find for the row of node $\Theta(u_1)$ of the classical partitioned system

$$\mathbf{K}_{\Theta(u_1),F(u_1)} \cdot \mathbf{d}_{F(u_1)} = -\mathbf{K}_{\Theta(u_1),E(u_1)} \cdot \mathbf{d}_{E(u_1)}. \tag{5.30}$$

Substituting in dominant terms and indices, and seeing from a simulation that the prevailing products of two shape functions in $\mathbf{K}_{\Theta(u_1),F(u_1)}$ are positive, we arrive at

$$\Big[\underbrace{\mathbb{H}^{1111}}_{(+ve)} \underbrace{F_{11}}_{1} \underbrace{F_{11}}_{1} \underbrace{\underbrace{\Delta u_{1,1}}_{(\text{node } \Theta)} \underbrace{\delta u_{1,1}}_{(\text{free nodes})}}_{(+ve)}\Big] \cdot \left[\mathbf{d}_{F(u_1)}\right] = -\Big[\underbrace{\mathbb{H}^{1111}}_{(+ve)} \underbrace{F_{11}}_{1} \underbrace{F_{11}}_{1} \underbrace{\underbrace{\Delta u_{1,1}}_{(\text{node } \Theta)}}_{(-ve)} \underbrace{\underbrace{\delta u_{1,1}}_{(\text{Ess. nodes})}}_{(+ve)}\Big] \cdot \left[\underbrace{\mathbf{d}_{E(u_1)}}_{(+ve)}\right], \tag{5.31}$$

which simplifies to

$$\underbrace{\mathbf{K}_{\Theta(u_1),F(u_1)}}_{(+\mathrm{ve})} \cdot \mathbf{d}_{F(u_1)} = -\underbrace{\mathbf{K}_{\Theta(u_1),E(u_1)}}_{(-\mathrm{ve})} \cdot \underbrace{\mathbf{d}_{E(u_1)}}_{(+\mathrm{ve})} . \tag{5.32}$$

Evidently, in order for the classical equation system of Eq. (5.32) to be satisfied the majority of free nodes must solve to have positive displacements $\mathbf{d}_{F(u_1)} \stackrel{!}{=} +ve$, and thus the body stretches. The only difference in signs between the equilibriums of Eq. (5.28) and the classical version of Eq. (5.32) is the resulting sign of $\mathbf{K}_{FE}$. Furthermore, the important difference between Eq. (5.27) populating $K_{\Theta(a_1),E(u_1)}$ and Eq. (5.31) populating $K_{\Theta(u_1),E(u_1)}$ is the signs of $\Delta a_{\gamma 1}$ and $\Delta u_{1,1}$, respectively. For this tension beam example the largest weighted *Gauss* points that populate $\mathbf{K}_{FE}$ are those in-between the relevant interacting nodes, with the free nodes at lesser x-coordinates and the essential nodes at the maximum x-coordinate. Given the free nodes are at a lesser x-coordinate than the gauss points, we approximate the variant $\Delta u_{1,1}$ as a derivative shape function that is negative in that direction $\Delta u_{1,1} \rightarrow B_{1,1} < 0$; however, we approximate the variant $\Delta a_{\gamma 1}$ as a shape function that is positive in that direction $\Delta a_{\gamma 1} \rightarrow N_1 > 0$, because the shape functions are always positive, and thus we see the difference in sign.

The aforementioned one element tension beam example was simplified to exclude boundary micro-conditions, and in such a scenario we have already established in Section 5.1.2 directly from the equilibrium equation that the micro-director must contract for all positive material parameters. However, the important finding from the breakdown of the partitioned FEM system is that it provides an explanation as to why boundary micro-conditions will not fix the problem of micro-director contracting for Sansour's micromorphic model. If we were to add a stretching essential boundary micro-condition $\mathbf{d}_{E(a_1)} = +ve$, as was done in the example of Figure 5.5b, we also find that $K_{F(a_1),E(a_1)} = +ve$ as it uses two positive shape functions, and hence the system of Eq. (5.28) will still only be satisfied with negative micro-director deformations (contracting).

The author previously motivated that not having strain gradient based micro-director strain in Eq. (5.22) causes spurious micro-director deformations, or contractions in this example, and that rather having strain gradient based micro-director strain would be more appropriate for a material with continuously connected fibres. The analysis of the partitioned FEM system served as additional evidence to support this hypothesis, as we can now see that if the relevant sections of the micromorphic $\mathbf{K}_{FE}$ can be made positive, it should be possible to achieve positive micro-director deformations (stretching) for a body under tension. Furthermore, the breakdown of constituting terms motivated that the relevant sections of the micromorphic $\mathbf{K}_{FE}$ would be made positive by changing the dominant micromorphic variant from $\Delta a_{\gamma r}$ to instead be $\Delta a_{\gamma r,i}$, i.e. strain gradient based. In turn, this would allow for approximations based on derivative shape functions instead of shape functions, which for the tension beam should result in micro-director stretching instead of contracting. In order to achieve this, the micromorphic formulation would need to be reworked, and thus the author developed an alternative micromorphic formulation to have the dominant micro-director strain measure as strain gradient based, and not deformation based in Sansour's micromorphic model. This alternative micromorphic formulation, named the MDO model, was previously introduced in Section 4.2 and is now explored in the following Section 5.3.

## 5.3 Alternative MDO micromorphic approach

The discussion of micro-director deformation behaviour in Section 5.2 highlighted possible issues with Sansour's version of the micromorphic model, which was attributed to the use of displacement based strain measures rather than gradient based strain measures. it is the opinion of the author that in order for the micromorphic model to correctly depict a fibrous material under tension, it should follow that the components of the stress measures are positive $\mathbf{S}^{(0)}, \mathbf{S}^{(1)}, \mathbf{S}^{(2)} > 0$ in the direction of the prescribed stretch $\bar{\mathbf{u}}$. This could still be achieved using a non-zero micro-boundary force or displacement, however, a different micromorphic model would need to be formulated. The author thus developed an alternative micromorphic formulation founded on strain gradient based micro-director strain. The reader is referred back to Section 4.2 for the derivations of this gradient based method, referred to as the MDO model henceforth.

The advantage of this MDO model over Sansour's model is that, for the volume integral in the variational formulation of Eq. (4.60), *Gauss*' divergence theorem can still be used on all of the terms acting on the micro-scale degrees of freedom, which was shown to not apply to the dominant terms of Sansour's model in Eq. (5.22). The reason for this is that for the MDO model only contains micro-director strain gradients in its mixed-scale and micro-scale strain measures, and thus the subsequent variant term in the volume integral of Eq. (4.60) is strain gradient based $\delta a_{\alpha r,l}$, instead of deformation based $\delta a_{\alpha r}$ for the dominant terms in Sansour's model. For the homogeneous deformation tension beam example of Section 5.1, but instead using the MDO model, if we were to take a perpendicular cut $\partial\mathcal{B}_x$ through the tension beam's length (x-axis) at any point, and after applying *Gauss*' divergence theorem to Eq. (4.60) to produce a surface integral representing the internal force acting normal to $\partial\mathcal{B}_x$ on the micro-scale degrees of freedom, in the absence of body forces, and with the external micro-traction $\hat{q}^{(\mathbf{n})}_{\alpha r}$ on the opposite end that keeps the divided member in equilibrium, we arrive at the following energy balance over micro-scale degrees of freedom

$$\frac{1}{2}\int_{\delta\mathcal{B}_x}\left[\zeta^\alpha \breve{S}^{(1)kl}F_{rk}+\zeta^\alpha \breve{S}^{(1)lk}F_{rk}+2\,\zeta^\beta\zeta^\alpha \breve{S}^{(2)ml}a_{\beta r,m}\right]n_l\delta a_{\alpha r}\;dA-\int_{\delta\mathcal{B}_{\mathcal{N}}}\hat{q}^{(\mathbf{n})}_{\alpha r}\delta a_{\alpha r}\;dA=0\,. \quad (5.33)$$

In the case of homogenous deformation, the surface area $A$ of $\partial\mathcal{B}_x$ is the same no matter where the cut along the x-axis is taken, because the cross-section dimensions are the same everywhere, and hence

$$\int_{\delta\mathcal{B}}\left([\frac{1}{2}\zeta^\alpha \breve{S}^{(1)kl}F_{rk}+\frac{1}{2}\zeta^\alpha \breve{S}^{(1)lk}F_{rk}+\zeta^\beta\zeta^\alpha \breve{S}^{(2)ml}a_{\beta r,m}]n_l-\hat{q}^{(\mathbf{n})}_{\alpha r}\right)\delta a_{\alpha r}\;dA=0, \quad (5.34)$$

and since $\delta\mathbf{a}_\alpha$ is a free variation, we find that at any perpendicular cross-section $\partial\mathcal{B}_x$ in the member

$$\left[\frac{1}{2}\zeta^\alpha \breve{S}^{(1)kl}F_{rk}+\frac{1}{2}\zeta^\alpha \breve{S}^{(1)lk}F_{rk}+\zeta^\beta\zeta^\alpha \breve{S}^{(2)ml}a_{\beta r,m}\right]n_l=\hat{q}^{(\mathbf{n})}_{\alpha r}. \quad \text{(Homog. def.)} \quad (5.35)$$

In the absence of a boundary micro-traction $\hat{q}^{(\mathbf{n})}_{\alpha 1}$, the same issue of opposing signs for the mixed-scale and micro-scale stresses in Sansour's model discussed in Section 5.2 persists here for the MDO model, whereby $\breve{S}^{(1)\alpha 1} \propto -\breve{S}^{(2)\alpha\alpha}$. It is worth noting as a side remark that the use of gradient based strain in the MDO model allows for negative micro-scale stresses $\breve{S}^{(2)\alpha\alpha} < 0$ even for micro-director stretching, so long as the micro-director strain gradient is negative. The crucial difference with the MDO model in Eq. (5.35) is that when there is indeed a tensile boundary micro-traction, it is now possible to have both positive stress measures $\breve{S}^{(1)\alpha 1}, \breve{S}^{(2)\alpha\alpha} > 0$. Furthermore, we have shown that this must be satisfied at all cross-sections of the beam due to *Gauss*' divergence theorem, and not just in the overall volume integral as with Sansour's model in Eq. (5.22). This is best illustrated by comparing the uniform MDO model stresses at *Gauss points* along the beam's axis in Figure 5.8, against Sansour's model stress in Figure 5.6.

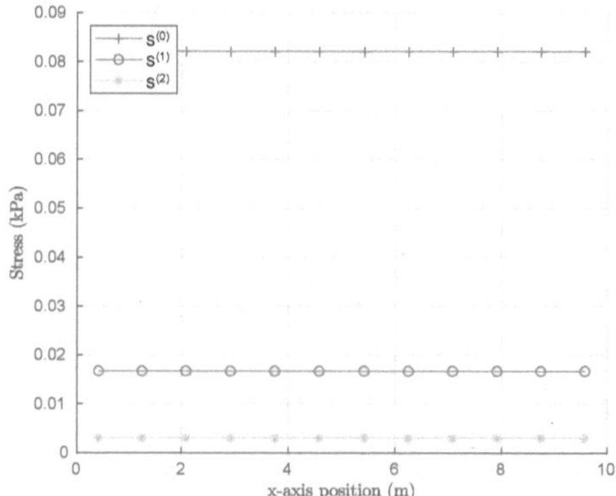


Fig. 5.8: Homogeneous deformation tension beam example: Graph of MDO model stresses at *Gauss points* along beam's axis for tensile boundary macro-traction $\hat{t}_1^{(\mathbf{n})} = 0.1\,\mathrm{kPa}$, and tensile boundary micro-traction $\hat{q}_{\gamma 1}^{(\mathbf{n})} = 0.02\,\mathrm{kPa}$ on free end (right face). We note that $S^{(0)11} + S^{(1)\gamma 1} = \hat{t}_1^{(\mathbf{n})}$, at all points in the beam. Additionally, we find $S^{(1)\gamma 1} + S^{(2)\gamma\gamma} = \hat{q}_{\gamma 1}^{(\mathbf{n})}$, which was not achieved using Sansour's model in Figure 5.6.

The ability of the MDO model to allow for micro-director stretching in the tension beam example, when all material parameters are positive for various boundary micro-tractions, is visible in Figure 5.9a. The example uses the linear constitutive equations of Eq. (4.66) for the macro-scale and Eq. (4.73) for the mixed-scale and micro-scale, and has a prescribed zero boundary micro-deformation $\bar{\mathbf{w}}_\gamma = \mathbf{0}$ on the member's fixed end. Furthermore, because the strain measures is strain gradient based, it enforces continuity between adjacent nodes, and thus the relative micro-director deformation is uniform no-matter the boundary micro-traction, as seen in Figure 5.9b. The author was not able to achieve these result using Sansour's model in this study, as per Section 5.2.

It is evident in Figure 5.9a that if a sufficiently large boundary micro-traction is applied, it is possible to achieve positive micro-director deformations using the author's MDO model. As such, the afore-mentioned requirement of $\mathbf{S}^{(0)}, \mathbf{S}^{(1)}, \mathbf{S}^{(2)} > 0$ in the direction of the prescribed stretch $\mathbf{u}$ is satisfied, which the author believes motivates that the MDO model represents the physical scenario of a fibrous tension beam realistically. Having achieved micro-director stretching for bulk material stretching with strictly positive material parameters, the author posed a new question: what is the minimum boundary micro-traction required to achieve the desired micro-director stretching, and how does that boundary micro-traction relate to the boundary macro-conditions? To answer this question, we continue from Eq. (5.35), and exploit the symmetry of $\check{\mathbf{S}}^{(1)}$, to give

$$\zeta^\alpha \check{S}^{(1)kl} F_{rk} n_l + \zeta^\alpha \zeta^\beta \check{S}^{(2)kl} a_{\beta r,k} n_l = \hat{q}_{\alpha r}^{(\mathbf{n})}. \tag{5.36}$$

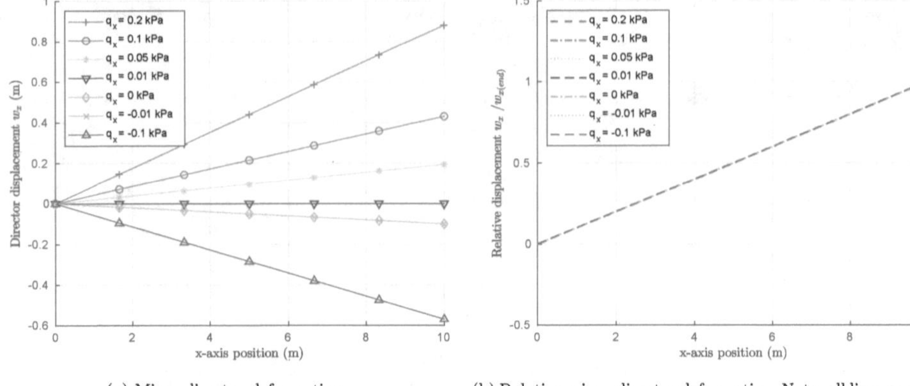


(a) Micro-director deformation.

(b) Relative micro-director deformation. Note: all lines overlap.

Fig. 5.9: Homogeneous deformation tension beam example for the MDO model: micro-boundary force $\hat{\mathbf{q}}^{(\mathbf{n})}_{\alpha}$ influence on micro-director deformation along the beam length for prescribed macro-stretch $\lambda =$ 1.01, and macro-scale linear isotropic material parameters $a_0 = 6$ kPa and $b_0 = 15$ kPa, and linear mixed-scale and micro-scale material parameters $A_1 = A_2 = 1$ kPa.

Next we substitute the stresses with the *Green* strain and material parameters from the strain energy functions of Eq. (4.73), such that $\breve{\mathbf{S}}^{(i)} = A_i \breve{\mathbf{E}}^{(i)}$, and hence

$$\zeta^{\alpha} A_1 \breve{E}^{(1)kl} F_{rk} n_l + \zeta^{\alpha}\zeta^{\beta} A_2 \breve{E}^{(2)kl} a_{\beta r,k} n_l = \hat{q}^{(\mathbf{n})}_{\alpha r}. \tag{5.37}$$

We now substitute the right *Cauchy-Green* strain using $\breve{\mathbf{E}}^{(i)} = 1/2(\breve{\mathbf{C}}^{(i)} - \breve{\mathbf{C}}^{(i)0})$ of Eq. (4.42)-(4.44) to give

$$\frac{1}{2}\zeta^{\alpha} A_1 \left(a_{\alpha s,k} F_{sl} + a_{\alpha s,l} F_{sk} - 2\delta_{kl}\right) F_{rk} n_l + \frac{1}{2} A_2 \zeta^{\alpha}\zeta^{\beta} \left(a_{\alpha s,k} a_{\beta s,l} - \delta_{kl}\right) a_{\beta r,k} n_l = \hat{q}^{(\mathbf{n})}_{\alpha r}. \tag{5.38}$$

For the tension beam example with homogeneous deformation, the only significant terms are those in the axis of prescribed deformation: $F_{11} = \lambda$; $a_{1,1}$; and $q^{(\mathbf{n})}_{\alpha 1}$, and after substituting these terms we arrive at

$$A_2 \zeta^{\alpha}\zeta^{\beta} a^3_{1,1} + 2\zeta^{\alpha} A_1 \lambda^2 a_{1,1} - \zeta^{\alpha}\zeta^{\beta} A_2 a_{1,1} - 2\zeta^{\alpha} A_1 \lambda = 2\hat{q}^{(\mathbf{n})}_{\alpha 1}. \tag{5.39}$$

The critical minimum boundary micro-traction required to ensure all strain and stress measures are positive occurs when there are zero micro-director displacements $w_{\alpha 1} = 0$, as was evident in Figure 5.9a, because as soon as $w_{\alpha 1} > 0$ all strains and stresses become positive. Therefore, for the special case of $w_{\alpha 1} = 0$ along the member, we find $a_{1,1} = 1$, and thus Eq. (5.39) simplifies to

$$\zeta^{\alpha} A_1 \left(\lambda^2 - \lambda\right) = \hat{q}^{(\mathbf{n})}_{\alpha 1}. \qquad \text{(critical micro-boundary force)} \tag{5.40}$$

Finally, we deduce that the critical minimum micro-boundary force $q^{(\mathbf{n})}_{\alpha r}$ depends on the macro-scale deformation gradient $\mathbf{F}$, the mixed-scale material parameter $A_1$, and the MDO micro-length $\zeta^{\alpha}$. In the case of the simulation example used in this section, where $A_1 = 1$, $\zeta^{\alpha} = 1$, and the prescribed macro-boundary displacement giving $\lambda = F_{11} = 1.01$, we find Eq. (5.40) reduces to

$q_{\alpha 1}^{(\mathbf{n})} = 1.01^2 - 1.01 = 0.0101$. This micro-boundary force applied to the MDO simulation produced the anticipated result of $w_{\alpha 1} = 0$, and thus confirms the proof. The preceding proof is only directly used for a macro-scale displacement-driven model, where $\lambda$ is prescribed. In the case of a macro-scale force-driven model where $t_{\alpha 1}^{(\mathbf{n})}$ is known, we can calculate $\lambda$ from the macro-equilibrium of Eq. (4.64) by substituting for the special case of $w_{\alpha 1} = 0$ such that $a_{1,1} = 1$. Once we solve for $\lambda$, we can then substitute $\lambda$ into Eq. (5.40) to find the required critical micro-traction $\hat{q}_{\alpha r}^{(\mathbf{n})}$.

The need for a boundary micro-condition would seem logical because the total force $\mathbf{f}_{tot}$ applied at the boundary of a fibrous material would generally be split between a portion of force applied through the bulk material ($\hat{\mathbf{t}}^{(\mathbf{n})}$) and the portion of force applied through the fibres ($\hat{\mathbf{q}}_{\alpha}^{(\mathbf{n})}$), such that $\mathbf{f}_{tot} = \hat{\mathbf{t}}^{(\mathbf{n})} A + \hat{\mathbf{q}}_{\alpha}^{(\mathbf{n})} A$. If the MDO model were to be used further, the attributing of boundary forces between the bulk material and the fibres would require consideration to ensure it reflects the physical system, and to calibrate the reorientations of the micro-directors as the fibres in the material.

In summary, the author formulated the MDO model and was able to achieve micro-director stretching in a tension beam using micro-boundary conditions and for strictly positive material parameters, which was not achieved in this study using Sansour's model. Furthermore, the author devised a novel proof for predicting the critical minimum boundary micro-traction required to achieve micro-director stretching. The potential drawback with the MDO model is that it must have some form of boundary micro-condition, otherwise the model does not solve. This aspect of the MDO model renders it more complicated for use in cardiac modelling, given the complexity of applying realistic boundary micro-conditions to the geometries of the heart. Conversely, it could be questioned whether it is physical to have a system that solves without the need for micro-boundary conditions, but that discussion is beyond the scope of this work. The fact that Sansour's model does not require boundary micro-conditions means it more easily applied to cardiac modelling, and as such it shall be used instead of the MDO model for the remaining modelling in this study. It is hoped that with more time and resources, the capabilities of the MDO model can be explored in cardiac modelling in future work.

## 5.4 Natural basis vector conversion issue

In the process of implementing the micromorphic model an interesting numerical limitation was uncovered inadvertently, whereby the following proposed method to convert mixed-scale terms from natural basis vectors to Cartesian basis vectors was found to be invalid for only one micro-director. The author determined the cause of the problem and developed the following explanation. The finding is included in this book in the spirit of academic transparency in the hope that the problem can be avoided by others, and because considerable time was spent uncovering the issue.

The generalized micromorphic variational formulation set out in Section 4.3 uses generalized basis vectors, or natural bases. In order to make the model implementation into the in-house modelling software SESKA less time consuming, it was decided at the outset that existing implementations of Cartesian based constitutive law and stress measures from classical models in SESKA could be reused with minor adjustments. However, the decision to use Cartesian based implementation requires a conversion of the strain measures from the natural bases seen Eq. (4.30)-Eq. (4.34) to Cartesian basis vectors. Finally, the Cartesian stresses are converted back to natural bases, so that it can be inserted back into the variational formulation. Note, the conversions are not necessary, but were only needed in order to reuse Cartesian based implementation.

The aforementioned mixed-scale conversion issue affects strain and stress in the same way, but the following demonstration is notated with stress $\tilde{S}^{(1)}_{r\gamma}$. The attempted conversions between natural bases and Cartesian bases were devised from Eq. (1.224) of Holzapfel (2000), which states that for general bases $\mathbf{g}_j \otimes \mathbf{g}^j = \mathbb{I}$, and hence

$$\mathbf{g}^r = (\mathbf{e}_i \otimes \mathbf{e}_i)\ \mathbf{g}^r = (\mathbf{g}^r \cdot \mathbf{e}_i)\,\mathbf{e}_i \tag{5.41}$$

$$\mathbf{e}_i = (\mathbf{g}^r \otimes \mathbf{g}_r)\ \mathbf{e}_i = (\mathbf{g}_r \cdot \mathbf{e}_i)\ \mathbf{g}^r. \tag{5.42}$$

Therefore, the natural bases stresses were converted to Cartesian stresses using Eq. (5.41)-(5.42) for $\tilde{\mathbf{G}}^r$ and $\tilde{\mathbf{I}}^\gamma$, which gave

$$\begin{aligned}
&\tilde{S}^{(1)}_{r\gamma}\left(\tilde{\mathbf{G}}^r \otimes \tilde{\mathbf{I}}^\gamma + \tilde{\mathbf{I}}^\gamma \otimes \tilde{\mathbf{G}}^r\right) \quad \text{(Natural)} && (5.43)\\
=\ &\tilde{S}^{(1)}_{r\gamma}\left((\tilde{\mathbf{G}}^r \cdot \mathbf{e}_i)\,\mathbf{e}_i \otimes (\tilde{\mathbf{I}}^\gamma \cdot \mathbf{e}_j)\,\mathbf{e}_j + (\tilde{\mathbf{I}}^\gamma \cdot \mathbf{e}_i)\,\mathbf{e}_i \otimes (\tilde{\mathbf{G}}^r \cdot \mathbf{e}_j)\,\mathbf{e}_j\right) && (5.44)\\
=\ &\tilde{S}^{(1)}_{r\gamma}\left[(\tilde{\mathbf{G}}^r \cdot \mathbf{e}_i)(\tilde{\mathbf{I}}^\gamma \cdot \mathbf{e}_j) + (\tilde{\mathbf{I}}^\gamma \cdot \mathbf{e}_i)(\tilde{\mathbf{G}}^r \cdot \mathbf{e}_j)\right]\mathbf{e}_i \otimes \mathbf{e}_j && (5.45)\\
=\ &\tilde{S}^{(1)}_{ij}\,\mathbf{e}_i \otimes \mathbf{e}_j \quad \text{(Cartesian).} && (5.46)
\end{aligned}$$

Once the Cartesian based implementation had transformed strain to stress, the process of converting the Cartesian stress back to natural bases stress was attempted by exploiting

$$\tilde{S}^{(1)}_{ij}\,\mathbf{e}_i \otimes \mathbf{e}_j = \frac{1}{2}\tilde{S}^{(1)}_{ij}\,(\mathbf{e}_i \otimes \mathbf{e}_j + \mathbf{e}_i \otimes \mathbf{e}_j) \quad \text{(Cartesian).} \tag{5.47}$$

The Cartesian bases were converted back to natural bases using Eq. (5.41)-(5.42) for $\tilde{\mathbf{G}}^r$ and $\tilde{\mathbf{I}}^\gamma$, which gave

$$= \frac{1}{2}\tilde{S}^{(1)}_{ij}\left((\tilde{\mathbf{G}}_t \cdot \mathbf{e}_i)\tilde{\mathbf{G}}^t \otimes (\tilde{\mathbf{I}}_\lambda \cdot \mathbf{e}_j)\tilde{\mathbf{I}}^\lambda + (\tilde{\mathbf{I}}_\lambda \cdot \mathbf{e}_i)\tilde{\mathbf{I}}^\lambda \otimes (\tilde{\mathbf{G}}_t \cdot \mathbf{e}_j)\tilde{\mathbf{G}}^t\right) \quad \text{(Natural).} \tag{5.48}$$

This was how the implementation was constructed; however, the model did not solve correctly, but it was not clear why. After substantial investigation, the author noted the following restrictions to $\mathbf{g}_j \otimes \mathbf{g}^j = \mathbb{I}$ from Eq. (1.224) of Holzapfel (2000), which had formed the basis of Eq. (5.41)-(5.42). For a three-dimensional macro-space and a three-dimensional micro-space (three micro-directors), we find the following

$$\left(\tilde{\mathbf{G}}_t \otimes \tilde{\mathbf{G}}^t\right) = \mathbb{I} \quad \& \quad \left(\tilde{\mathbf{I}}_\lambda \otimes \tilde{\mathbf{I}}^\lambda\right) = \mathbb{I} \quad (t = \lambda = 1, 2, 3), \tag{5.49}$$

and thus the conversion from Eq. (5.43) to Eq. (5.46) would be valid. However, for a three-dimensional macro-space with only a one-dimensional micro-space, we find the following problem

$$\left(\tilde{\mathbf{I}}_\lambda \otimes \tilde{\mathbf{I}}^\lambda\right) \neq \mathbb{I} \qquad (\lambda = 1, \text{ and 3D macro-space}). \tag{5.50}$$

The statement of Eq. (5.50) would be valid for a truly one-dimensional space; however, the micro-director has degrees of freedom in three-dimensional space. For example, let us assume a one-dimensional micro-space in which $\mathbf{a}^0 = \mathbf{e}_1$, and from Eq. (4.23) we find $\tilde{\mathbf{I}}_\lambda = \mathbf{a}^0 = \mathbf{e}_1$. We thus prove Eq. (5.50) as follows

$$\begin{aligned}
&\tilde{\mathbf{I}}_\lambda \cdot \tilde{\mathbf{I}}^\lambda = \mathbf{e}_1 \cdot \tilde{\mathbf{I}}^\lambda = 1 \quad \because \left(\tilde{\mathbf{I}}_\lambda \cdot \tilde{\mathbf{I}}^\gamma = \delta^{\cdot\gamma}_{\lambda}\right) && (5.51)\\
\therefore\ &\tilde{\mathbf{I}}^\lambda = \mathbf{e}_1 && (5.52)\\
&\left(\tilde{\mathbf{I}}_\lambda \otimes \tilde{\mathbf{I}}^\lambda\right) = (\mathbf{e}_1 \otimes \mathbf{e}_1) \neq \mathbb{I}, \qquad (\lambda = 1, \tilde{\mathbf{I}}_\lambda = \tilde{\mathbf{I}}^\lambda = \mathbf{e}_1). && (5.53)
\end{aligned}$$

As such, the conversion from Eq. (5.43) to Eq. (5.46) would be invalid. It is typically valid for curvilinear basis vectors to use the aforementioned property $\mathbb{I} = \mathbf{g}_j \otimes \mathbf{g}^j$ from Eq. (1.224) of Holzapfel (2000); however, the author has shown that it is not valid to use this property when representing a one-dimensional space $\mathcal{S}(1)$ using a single curvilinear basis vector that has degrees of freedom in three-dimensional space $\mathbb{E}(3)$. The property is only valid when the number $(m)$ of dimensions of the micro-space $\mathcal{S}(m)$ compliments the number of dimensions of the macro-space $\mathbb{E}(m)$. For the three-dimensional macro-space $\mathbb{E}(3)$ example of this section, the property would only be valid for a three-dimensional micro-space $\mathcal{S}(3)$, and only then could this proposed method of bases conversion be used correctly. Similarly, for a two-dimensional macro-space $\mathbb{E}(2)$ example, a two-dimensional micro-space $\mathcal{S}(2)$ is required for valid bases conversions using this property.

## 5.5 Strain-dependent anisotropy

The micromorphic model is capable of describing strain-dependent anisotropy, which is useful for cardiac modelling as muscle fibres respond dominantly for small strains while the ECM responds dominantly for large strains [21, 26]. This section will examine the strain-dependent anisotropy of the micromorphic model using the examples of a tension beam and a perforated plate, as both bodies exhibit anisotropy over small strains but exhibit isotropy over larger strains. The myocardium does not exhibit isotropy over larger strains, however, an isotropic response is used in these examples to demonstrate strain-dependent material behaviour most transparently.

### 5.5.1 Tension beam example

von Hoegen et al. (2017) adapted the example used by Himpel et al. (2008) of a tension beam - with angled fibres at 30 degrees to the beam's axis as seen in Figure 5.10a - to highlight the capabilities of the micromorphic model over the classical model. The findings of von Hoegen et al. are hence reproduced in this section. The most basic micromorphic model was tested with the tension beam to ensure transparent representation of its mixed-scale and micro-scale effects. The isotropic strain energy function of Eq. (4.66) producing a linear material response was used for the macro-scale, as this ensures all anisotropic behaviour is attributed to the mixed-scale and micro-scale. Additionally, the strain energy functions of Eq. (4.73) producing a linear material response were used for the mixed-scale and micro-scale. The transversely isotropic strain energy $\psi_c$ producing a linear material response was chosen for the classical model, in order to also make the classical model behaviour as transparent as possible

$$\psi_c = \frac{1}{2} A_c Q, \tag{5.54}$$

where $A_c$ is a stress scaling material parameter, and the orthotropic function $Q$ of Usyk et al. (2002) introduced in Section 3.5 in Eq. (3.28) was adapted to produce transversely isotropic material behaviour by giving two of the preferred material directions equal material parameters as follows

$$b_{ss} = b_{nn} \quad \text{and} \quad b_{fn} = b_{fs}. \tag{5.55}$$

The material parameters used for the micromorphic model and the classical model are given in Table 5.3, and were chosen to produce a high degree of transverse isotropy caused by the preferred material direction.

Table 5.3: Material parameters used in the tension beam example with both the classical model preferred material direction and the micromorphic micro-directors orientated at 30 degrees from the beam's axis.

| | $A_c$ | $b_{ff}$ | $b_{ss}$ | $b_{nn}$ | $b_{fs}$ | $b_{fn}$ | $b_{sn}$ |
|---|---|---|---|---|---|---|---|
| Classical | 0.3 | 152 | 7 | 7 | 2.5 | 2.5 | 3 |
| units | kPa | - | - | - | - | - | - |
| | $a_0$ | $b_0$ | $A_1$ | $A_2$ | | | |
| Micromorphic | 40 | 60 | 2400 | 2400 | | | |
| units | kPa | kPa | kPa | kPa | | | |

Simulations were run for various prescribed horizontal displacements $\bar{u}_x$ on $\partial\mathcal{B}_D$, and no boundary conditions regarding the micro-director. The behaviour of the micromorphic model compared with the classical model is seen in Figure 5.10, and it is clear that the micromorphic model allows for distinctly different deformations from the classical model. For smaller displacements both classical and micromorphic models exhibit significant anisotropy by deflecting downwards and produce almost identical deformations. For larger displacements the classical model deforms to an s-shape because of the preferred material direction, as anticipated by Himpel et al. (2008) for transverse isotropy. However, the micromorphic micro-directors can reorientate elastically to achieve an almost homogeneous elongation of the bulk material (in terms of $\mathbf{u}$) for larger deformations, which could only be achieved by Himpel et al. using an algorithm that forces the preferred material direction to align with the maximum strain direction as a dissipative reorientation.

The micromorphic model deformations are consistent with those produced by von Hoegen et al. (2017), and are pertinent because they confirm the capability of the micromorphic mixed-scale and micro-scale to replicate a strain-evolving material response for different ranges of deformation. This is particularly useful for cardiac modelling, because the muscle fibres account for much of the cardiac tissue stiffness at small strains, whereas the ECM dominates at large strains [26, 21].

### 5.5.2 Perforated plate example

The tension beam example of Section 5.5.1 was effective for demonstrating the contrast in deformations between the strain-dependent anisotropy of the micromorphic model and the conventional anisotropy of a classical model. The following perforated plate example confirms such differences for a more complex material geometry. The perforated plate has outward prescribed displacements $\bar{u}$ on $\partial\mathcal{B}_D$ on all four sides, and no micro-boundary conditions. The plate material has a preferred material direction or micromorphic micro-directors orientated at 45° from the horizontal as seen in Figure 5.11.

The same rudimentary linear constitutive laws of the tension beam example in Section 5.5.1 were again used for the perforated plate; namely the linear transversely isotropic constitutive law $\psi_c$ for the classical model, and the linear isotropic macro-scale with linear mixed-scale and micro-scale constitutive law for the micromorphic model. The versatility of the micromorphic model to vary the effect of strain-dependent anisotropy is highlighted by comparing stiffer micromorphic material parameters in the strain energy function (labelled with $\tilde{\psi}_1$) with more compliant micromorphic material parameters in the strain energy function (labelled with $\tilde{\psi}_2$). The material parameters for the three models tested are found in Table 5.4.

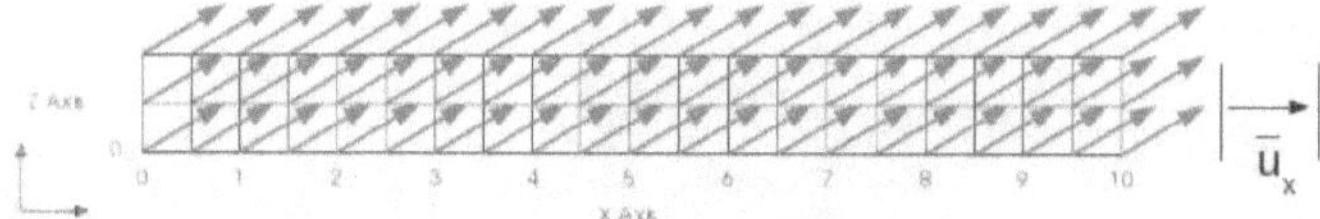


(a) The undeformed beam with classical anisotropy direction and micromorphic micro-directors orientated at 30° from the beam's axis.

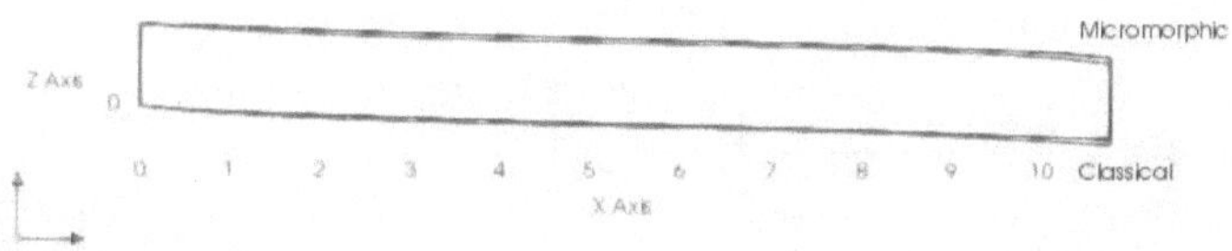


(b) Prescribed displacement - $\bar{u}_x = 0.75m$. Both classical (red) and micromorphic (blue) models exhibit significant anisotropy by deflecting downwards and produce almost identical deformations for smaller strain.

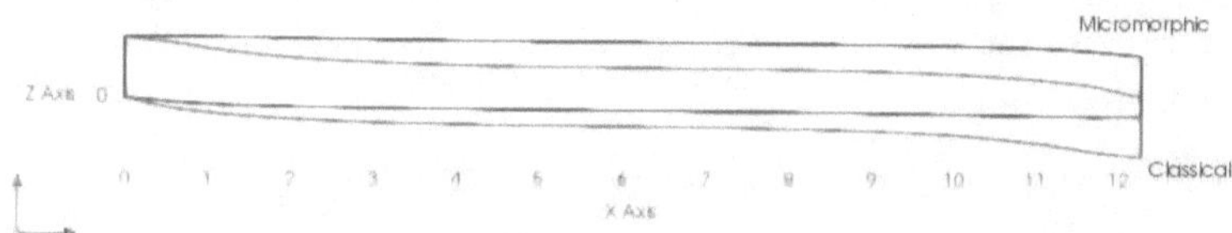


(c) Prescribed displacement - $\bar{u}_x = 2.25m$. The classical model (red) continues to show significant anisotropy, whereas the micromorphic model (blue) begins to deform isotropically.

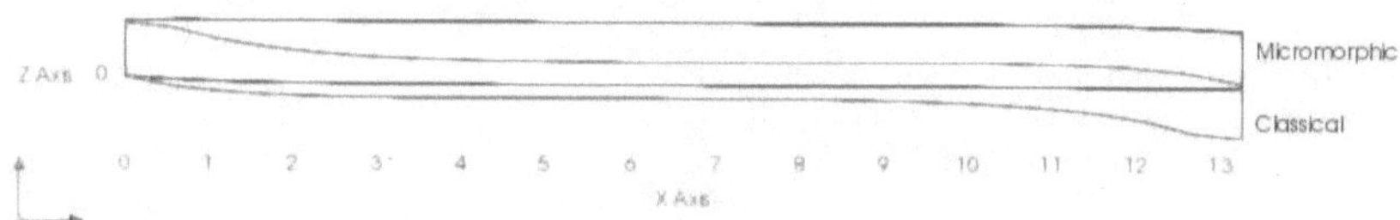


(d) Prescribed displacement - $\bar{u}_x = 3.25$. The classical model (red) at this larger strain shows severely anisotropic deformation, however, the micromorphic model (blue) has returned to near perfect isotropic deformation.

Fig. 5.10: Tension beam deformations for various prescribed horizontal displacements $\bar{u}_x$ on $\partial\mathcal{B}_D$ with the classical model preferred material direction and the micromorphic micro-directors both orientated at 30° above the beam's axis. The linear transversely isotropic classical model are shown in red, and those of the linear micromorphic model with an isotropic macro-scale are shown in blue.

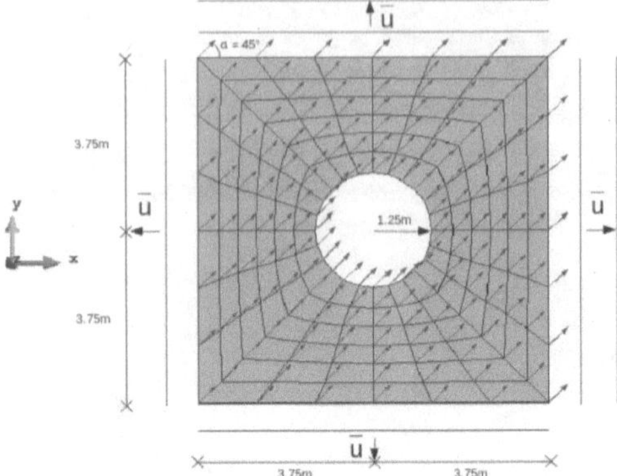


Fig. 5.11: Perforated plate example in its undeformed configuration with prescribed displacements $\bar{u}$ on $\partial\mathcal{B}_D$, and the classical model preferred material direction and the micromorphic micro-directors both orientated at 45° to the horizontal. The sides of the plate are 7.5 m $\times$ 7.5 m and the radius of the perforation is 1.25 m.

Table 5.4: Material parameters used for the perforated plate example.

| | $A_c$ | $b_{ff}$ | $b_{ss}$ | $b_{nn}$ | $b_{fs}$ | $b_{fn}$ | $b_{sn}$ |
|---|---|---|---|---|---|---|---|
| Classical ($\psi_c$) | 0.3 | 152 | 7 | 7 | 2.5 | 2.5 | 3 |
| units | kPa | - | - | - | - | - | - |
| | $a_m$ | $b_m$ | $A_1$ | $A_2$ | | | |
| Micromorphic ($\tilde{\psi}_1$) | 4 | 6 | 150 | 150 | | | |
| Micromorphic ($\tilde{\psi}_2$) | 4 | 6 | 50 | 50 | | | |
| units | kPa | kPa | kPa | kPa | | | |

The deformations of the three models are shown in Figure 5.12. For the smaller displacement condition of $\bar{u} = 1.0$ m we find non-uniform deformations from the classical transversely isotropic model in Figure 5.12e, and from the stiffer micromorphic model in Figure 5.12a. In contrast, the subtly non-uniform deformations of the more compliant micromorphic model are seen in Figure 5.12c, thus demonstrating how the extent of anisotropy can be manipulated as required. The deformation of the classical model at $\bar{u} = 3.0$ m remains visibly anisotropic in Figure 5.12f, as expected. However, both micromorphic models are able to return to an isotropic deformation (circular perforation) at larger deformations as seen in Figure 5.12b and Figure 5.12d. The explanation for this changing behaviour at larger strains is attributed to reorientations of the micro-directors such that the strain energy is minimized. For the geometry of the hole plate subjected to biaxial tension, the minimized energy state is that of a radial symmetric micro-director orientation [90], as seen by the circumferential deformations of the micro-directors in Figure 5.13. The largest micro-director deformations occur where the magnitude of the angle between the radial macro-displacements and the initial micro-director orientation is greatest, as the micro-directors must deform to orientate radially.

Once more, the micromorphic results produced by von Hoegen et al. (2017) were successfully corroborated in this study. The evidence of anisotropy at smaller strains followed with isotropy at larger strain achieved from elastic deformation by the micromorphic model promotes its potential usefulness and suitability for cardiac modelling. Biological tissues generally comprise of a network of components - each with unique stiffness contributions varying at different strain magnitudes. The sophisticated material response of strain-dependent anisotropy was only achieved with classical models through algorithmic treatment and supplementary iterative techniques, such as the methods implemented by Himpel et al. (2008) or Fausten et al. (2016), and only for dissipative reorientation not elastic reorientation achieved with the micromorphic model.

In summary, this chapter has explored the fundamental behaviour of the micromorphic model to better grasp uniqueness of solutions for the model, and the effect of mixed-scale and micro-scale material parameters on the deformation of the micro-director and on the overall stiffness response of the material. Furthermore, the capability of the micromorphic model to exhibit strain-dependent anisotropy has been demonstrated. Equipped with an enhanced understanding of the micromorphic model, we now apply the micromorphic model to cardiac tissue modelling in Section 6.

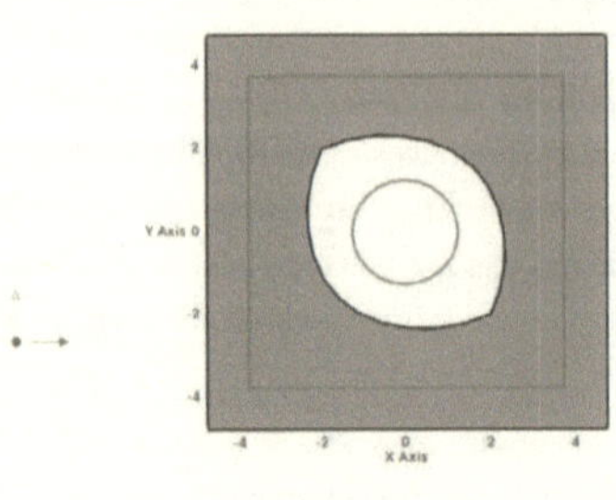


(a) Stiffer micromorphic model ($\tilde{\psi_1}$): $\bar{u} = 1.0$ m.

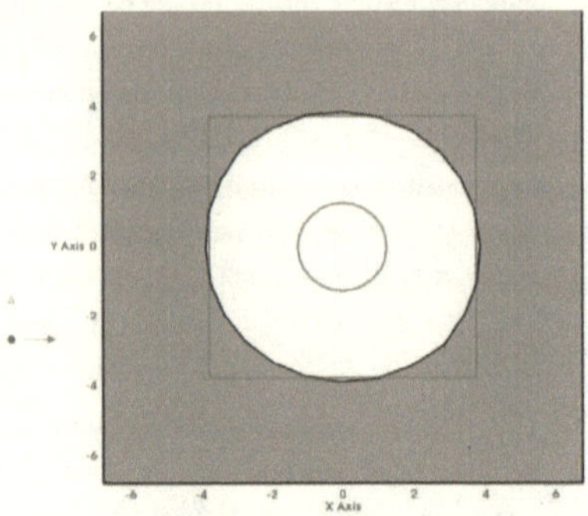


(b) Stiffer micromorphic model ($\tilde{\psi_1}$): $\bar{u} = 3.0$ m.

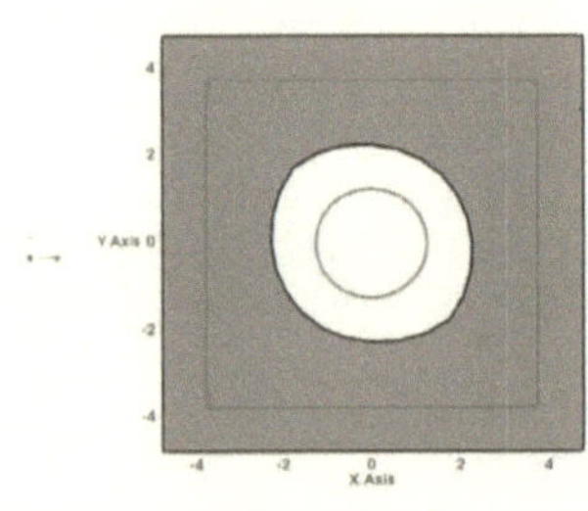


(c) Compliant micromorphic model ($\tilde{\psi_2}$): $\bar{u} = 1.0$ m.

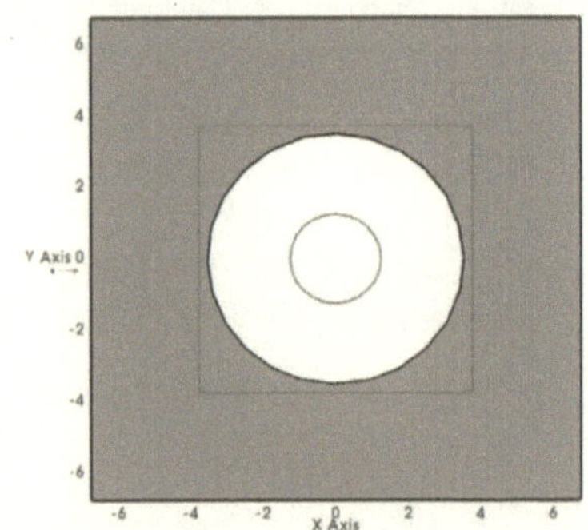


(d) Compliant micromorphic model ($\tilde{\psi_2}$): $\bar{u} = 3.0$ m.

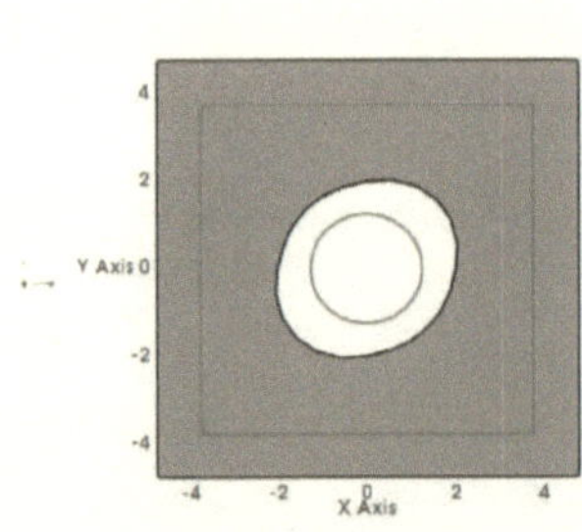


(e) Classical model ($\psi_c$): $\bar{u} = 1.0$ m.

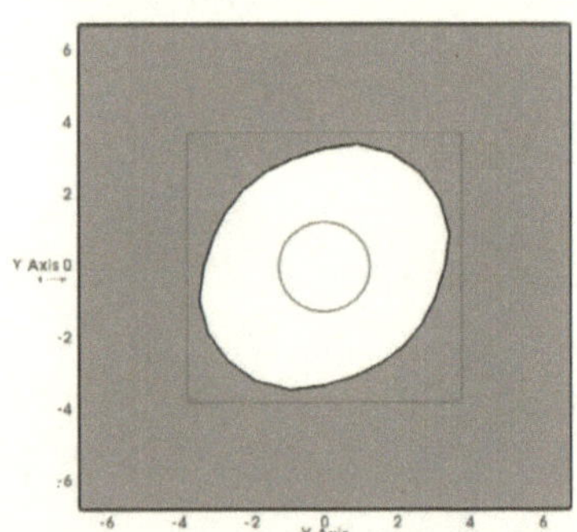


(f) Classical model ($\psi_c$): $\bar{u} = 3.0$ m.

Fig. 5.12: Perforated plate deformations for prescribed displacements $\bar{u}_x$ on $\partial\mathcal{B}_D$ using two micromorphic models and a classical transversely isotropic model. Undeformed preferred material direction and micromorphic micro-directors at 45° to the horizontal. The micromorphic model displays anisotropy at $\bar{u} = 1.0$ m, but then isotropy at $\bar{u} = 3.0$ m due to the reorientation of the micro-directors.

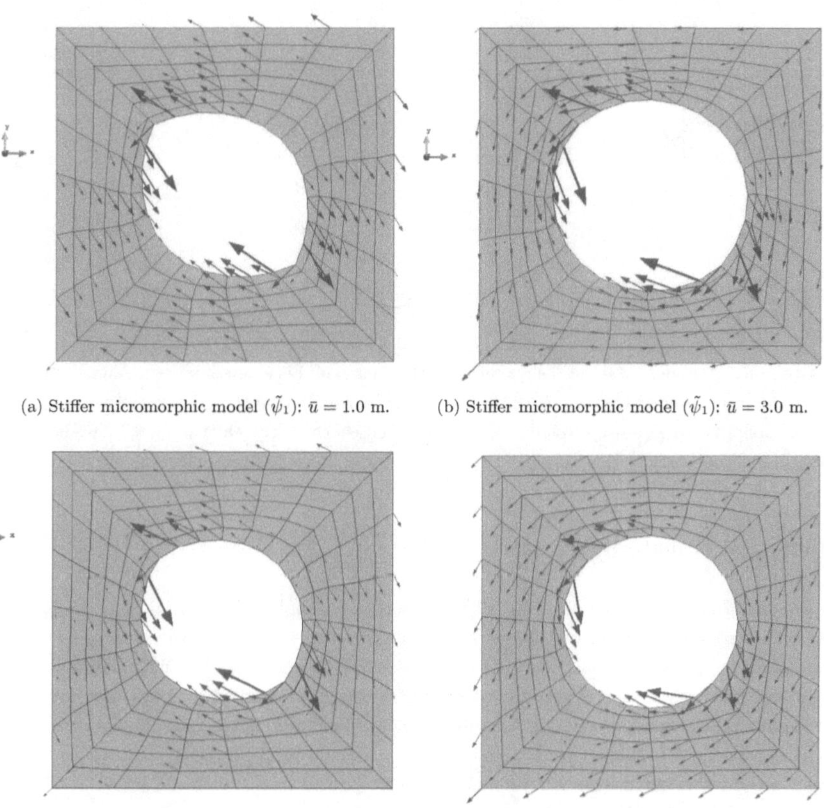

(a) Stiffer micromorphic model ($\tilde{\psi}_1$): $\bar{u} = 1.0$ m. (b) Stiffer micromorphic model ($\tilde{\psi}_1$): $\bar{u} = 3.0$ m.

(c) Compliant micromorphic model ($\tilde{\psi}_2$): $\bar{u} = 1.0$ m. (d) Compliant micromorphic model ($\tilde{\psi}_2$): $\bar{u} = 3.0$ m.

Fig. 5.13: Perforated plate micro-director displacements shown as blue vectors for prescribed displacements $\bar{u}_x$ on $\partial\mathcal{B}_D$ using a stiffer micromorphic model and a more compliant micromorphic model. Undeformed preferred material direction and micromorphic micro-directors at 45° to the horizontal. The micro-directors deform circumferentially to align radially in order to minimize the strain energy function, which is consistent with the results achieved by [90].

# 6

# Cardiac Models

The fundamental behaviour of Sansour's micromorphic model was assessed in Section 5. The model is now applied to cardiac models to assess the potential for the micromorphic micro-director to represent myocytes of the myocardium. The model will first be calibrated to triaxial shear experiments, and then further calibrated to a pressure-volume relationship. Subsequently, the passive filling phase of the left ventricle will be simulated using patient-specific geometry of the left ventricle.

## 6.1 Calibration of material parameters

The diastolic filling of the left ventricle can only be realistically simulated computationally once representative material parameters have been established for the strain energy function of the model. In the case of the proposed novel micromorphic constitutive law, it is necessary to find calibrated material parameters that can replicate the behaviour of heart tissue. The calibration procedures for complex non-linear FEM models are usually computationally expensive, in particular if there are many material parameters to calibrate such as in this micromorphic model, and therefore an efficient optimization algorithm is employed to facilitate the calibration process.

### 6.1.1 Bounded Levenberg-Marquardt (BLVM) optimization algorithm

The calibration of material parameters, known as an inverse problem, requires a search for a combination of material parameters that enable the numerical simulation to successfully approximate experimental data [10]. The optimization algorithms used for material parameter identification can be divided into two branches: gradient based algorithms [6] and non-gradient based algorithms [30]. The gradient based algorithms - such as the *steepest decent*, *Levenberg-Marquardt* or *Gauss-Newton* methods - achieve fastest convergence to a local minimum; however, they are not typically robust in finding the global minimum and are dependent on the initial parameters selected. In contrast, non-gradient based methods are superior at finding a solution to a global minimum from a larger parameter range; however, the convergence to the solution is slower than gradient-based methods.

The optimization algorithm used in this research is the *Bounded Levenberg-Marquardt* (BLVM) for least-squares curve fitting problems and is based on the work of Levenberg (1944) and Marquardt (1963). The method is referred to as bounded because the parameters are confined to acceptable ranges. The BLVM scheme was implemented by the Computational Continuum Mechanics (CCM)

Group of the University of Cape Town, which was adapted from the MATLAB script of Le Riche and Guyon (2000). Additionally, the scheme was supplemented in this study with simple error handling, assigning a large default error when the script reached divergent mixed-scale and micro-scale material parameter combinations to enable the script to continue its search without terminating. The cost function that must be minimized is formulated using the difference between the numerically simulated results and experimental data. The algorithm for the BLVM method is outlined in Figure 6.1.

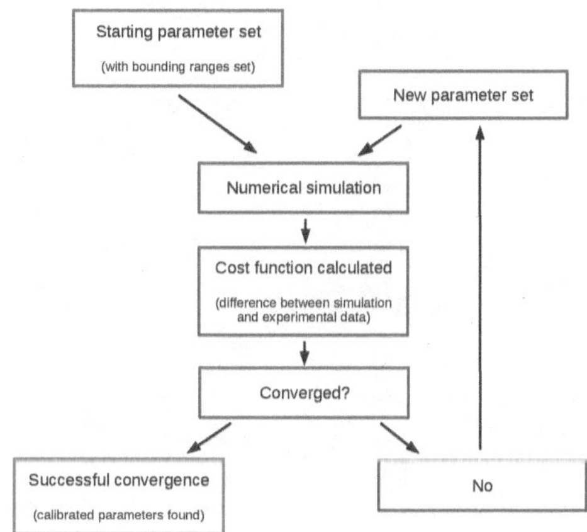


Fig. 6.1: Flowchart of the *Bounded Levenberg-Marquardt* (BLVM) algorithm used for the calibration of micromorphic model material parameters.

The cost function used by the algorithm was based upon the *sum of squared error* (SSE), which was converted into a *performance index* (PI) based upon the number of calibration experiments $m$, as per Eq. (6.1).

$$\mathrm{SSE} = \sum_{i=1}^{n} \left(x_{i(model)} - x_{i(data)}\right)^2; \qquad \mathrm{PI} = \frac{\mathrm{SSE}}{2m} \tag{6.1}$$

### 6.1.2 Triaxial shear experiments

The invasive nature of mechanically testing cardiac tissue has lead to a shortage of data on human samples. Until recently the experiment conducted by Dokos et al. (2002) on porcine cardiac tissue was considered a close substitute for human cardiac tissue, and was used by von Hoegen et al. (2016) to calibrate a similar micromorphic model. However, there is now data available for human cardiac tissue courtesy of the biaxial experiments [80] and subsequent triaxial shear tests by Sommer et al. (2015). The triaxial shear experiments involved shearing myocardial tissue sample along the 6 local fibre-specific planes, as seen in Figure 6.2, and were used for calibration in this study.

The results achieved by Sommer et al. are consistent with the porcine results of Dokos et al.; both found the two shear planes of FS and FN to be stiffest, with porcine tissue having as much as twice the stiffness of human tissue for those shear modes. Further, both studies found the shear planes of NF and NS to be most compliant. Hussan et al. (2012) were able to distinguish myocyte contributions in FN and FS modes, whereas NS and NF modes were attributed to the p-chain network of the ECM that bind myocytes together.

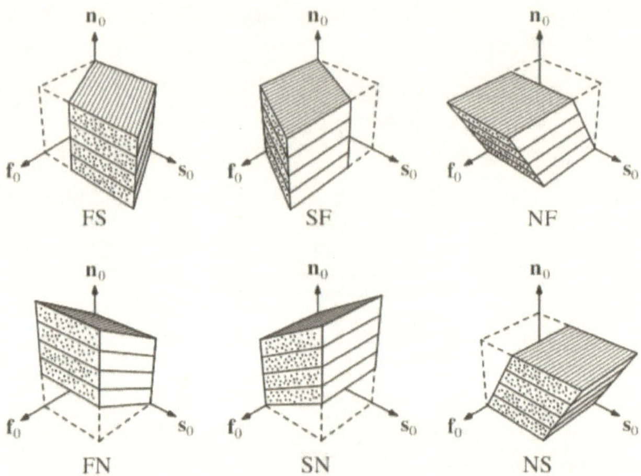


Fig. 6.2: Triaxial shear experiment: the 6 simple shear modes for a cube of myocardium tissue in terms of the tissue's local axes with respect to the muscle fibre $\mathbf{f}_0$, sheet $\mathbf{s}_0$, and the sheet-normal $\mathbf{n}_0$ directions [81].

The myocardium tissue cubes excised for the experiments performed by Sommer et al. were 4 mm $\times$ 4 mm $\times$ 4 mm in size. They investigated the micro-structure of the myocardium using second-harmonic generation (SHG) microscopy and were able to aggregate the dispersion of the fibre direction. The myocytes were found to rotate by $14.8° \pm 6.9°$ per $mm$ depth. The fibre dispersion for the calibration model with sides of $4mm$ was therefore calculated to total 60°, where the epicardium side of the cube was given an angle of $+30°$ and the endocardium an angle of $-30°$. The top and bottom surfaces of the cube were glued to plates, and the bottom surface was fixed while the top surface was sheared without any rotations allowed to the top and bottom surfaces. The boundary conditions applied to the cubes were such that $u_f = u_s = u_n = 0$ mm on the bottom surface, and only one non-zero displacement on the top surface, such as $u_f = 2$ mm and $u_s = u_n = 0$ mm for SF and NF modes. This achieved 0.5 shear strains, sufficient to show the non-linearity of the tissue's stiffness. No boundary conditions on the micro-director ($\mathbf{w}_D$) were prescribed, as further investigations into the consequence of micro-director boundary conditions are needed.

The micro-director internal length scale was set to $l_\alpha = 1 \times 10^{-6}$ m in order to render the higher-order contributions attributed to $\tilde{\mathbf{K}}_\alpha^{(i)}$ negligible, so that the micromorphic mixed-scale and micro-scale effects would be easier to interpret. The BLVM algorithm introduced in Section 6.1.1 was used to calibrate the macro-scale parameters $A_0, b_{ff}, b_{ss}, b_{nn}, b_{fs}, b_{fn}, b_{sn}$ from the non-linear orthotropic macro-scale strain energy function of Eq. (4.68) and Eq. (4.69), where the compressibility coefficient was fixed at $A_{comp} = 100$ kPa as per [79]. The mixed-scale and micro-scale material parameters of $A_1, B_1, A_2, B_2$ from the non-linear strain energy functions of Eq. (4.74) were also calibrated in this process. Convexity of the strain energy function is important and it needs to be positive definite [36, 92]; this was enforced by keeping all material parameters positive , except $B_1$ and $B_2$ which can be negative as they influence non-linearity only.

Even though the BLVM algorithm is relatively robust, it is still susceptible to converging to a local minimum, and not the global minimum of best fitting parameters, depending on what the starting material parameters are for the algorithm. The large number of material parameters in this model introduces the *curse of dimensionality* with respect to the choice of starting parameters for the calibration [2]. The problem is such that as the number of parameters increases, the number of starting points for calibrations grows exponentially if an exhaustive calibration is desired [64]. Furthermore, the interdependence of micro-parameters was proven in the numerical example of Section 5.5.1, and this further compounds the curse of dimensionality problem.

The risk of finding a local minimum solution was mitigated by choosing various starting parameter values for the algorithm, and a recurring global minimum was achieved to satisfy reasonable confidence in the calibrated solution. The calibrated material parameters for the micromorphic model ($\tilde{\psi}$) are found in Table 6.1, and it is worth noting that the result gave a near linear mixed/micro-scale constitutive law because $B_1 \approx B_2 \approx 0$.

Table 6.1: Calibrated material parameters from triaxial shear experiments on left ventricular muscle tissue for the micromorphic model ($\tilde{\psi}^{(0)}, \tilde{\psi}^{(1)}, \tilde{\psi}^{(2)}$), the equivalent macro-scale classical non-linear orthotropic model ($\psi^e$), and the classical non-linear orthotropic model ($\psi^c$) calibrated in Rama and Skatulla (2018).

| **Parameter** | **Value** | | | **Units** |
|---|---|---|---|---|
| macro-scale | $\tilde{\psi}^{(0)}$ | $e$ | $c$ | |
| $A_0$ | 0.284 | 0.284 | 0.19 | kPa |
| $A_{comp}$ | 100 | 100 | 100 | kPa |
| $b_{ff}$ | 21.03 | 21.03 | 23.92 | |
| $b_{ss}$ | 8.02 | 8.02 | 5.89 | |
| $b_{nn}$ | 0.22 | 0.22 | 0.59 | |
| $b_{fs}$ | 10.68 | 10.68 | 12.74 | |
| $b_{fn}$ | 8.12 | 8.12 | 10.19 | |
| $b_{sn}$ | 9.71 | 9.71 | 11.70 | |
| mixed-scale | $\tilde{\psi}^{(1)}$ | | | |
| $A_1$ | 26.72 | - | - | kPa |
| $B_1$ | 0.00 | - | - | |
| micro-scale | $\tilde{\psi}^{(2)}$ | | | |
| $A_2$ | 0.029 | - | - | kPa |
| $B_2$ | 0.0066 | - | - | |
| $l_\alpha$ | $1 \times 10^{-6}$ | - | - | m |

The calibration results can be seen in Figure 6.3, and the error performance index for the micromorphic model was PI $= 2.44 \times 10^{-3}$. The same shear experiment calibration was done by Rama and Skatulla (2018) using the classical non-linear orthotropic model ($\psi^c$) proposed by Usyk et al. and previously outlined in Section 3.5. Rama and Skatulla's results were also plotted on Figure 6.3, and it can be seen that the micromorphic model has improved the calibration over the classical model, particularly for the largest shear modes of FS and FN. However, it is noted that the shear mode of NS was not as close to the measured data. The classical model gave an error of PI $= 3.81 \times 10^{-3}$, and therefore the micromorphic calibration improved the performance index by 36%. The calibration appears better from a qualitative perspective than that achieved by the micromorphic model of von Hoegen et al. (2016) on similar porcine tissue shear experiments, particularly for shear modes FS and FN.

The effect of the mixed-scale and micro-scale in the micromorphic model was made visible by plotting the equivalent classical non-linear orthotropic model ($\psi^e$) in Figure 6.3, proposed by Usyk et al. and previously outlined in Section 3.5, using the same macro-scale material parameters of the micromorphic model. It is worth noting that it was confirmed in simulations that the micromorphic model gives the same results as the equivalent macro-scale classical model as the micro-parameters tend to zero: $A_1, A_2 \to 0$ kPa. However, it is not possible to run a model with $A_1, A_2 = 0$ kPa as the stiffness matrix is ill-formed. The gross difference and percentage difference in shear stress between the micromorphic model and equivalent macro-scale classical model can be seen in Figure 6.4a and Figure 6.4b, respectively. The percentage difference decreases with larger strain, which compliments the hypothesis that the motion of myocytes relative to the ECM is predominantly mobilized at smaller strains. For this set of material parameters the shear modes SF and SN are most influenced by the mixed-scale and micro-scale. However, it was observed that for other local minimum calibrations with different final mixed-scale and micro-scale material parameters, the mixed-scale and micro-scale could affect different combinations of shear modes. This should be investigated in future work to ensure the mixed-scale and micro-scale contributions match the actual contributions due to non-affine myocyte motion that have been experimentally determined once such data is available.

The larger contribution of the SN and SF shear modes is explained in part by the fact that the micro-director is activated and displaced, as seen in the magnitude of micro-director displacements $|\delta \mathbf{w}|$ in Figure 6.5. Conversely, shear modes FS and NS did not have a noticeable mixed-scale and micro-scale contributions and the micro-directors were barely displaced. It is not clear why the contributions from shear modes FN and NF were negligible, even though there were significant micro-director displacements. It is hypothesized by the author that those displacements are energy minimizing, such that it makes a minimum contribution to the boundary macro-traction vector $\hat{\mathbf{t}}^{(n)}$ in Eq. (4.57) through term $\tilde{S}^{(1)}_{j\beta} a_{\beta r}$, by displacing the micro-director $\mathbf{w}_\beta$ away (perpendicular) from the plane of macro-displacements $\mathbf{u}$, and hence nullifying its contribution.

The shear mode FS did not seem to have a noticeable mixed-scale and micro-scale contribution, which corroborates with the simple shear example of von Hoegen et al. (2017), and their explanation for this is now expanded upon by the author. For simple shear of $\partial u_2 / \partial X_1 = \gamma$ and fibres orientated such that $\mathbf{f}_0 = \mathbf{a}^0 = \mathbf{e}_1$, we find the right *Cauchy-Green* strain $\tilde{\mathbf{C}}^{(1)}$ with

$$\mathbf{F} = \begin{bmatrix} 1 & 0 & 0 \\ \gamma & 1 & 0 \\ 0 & 0 & 1 \end{bmatrix}, \qquad \mathbf{a} = \begin{bmatrix} 1 + w_1 \\ w_2 \\ w_3 \end{bmatrix}, \qquad \tilde{C}^{(1)0}_{j\beta} = \mathbf{I}^T \mathbf{a}^0 = \begin{bmatrix} 1 \\ 0 \\ 0 \end{bmatrix}, \tag{6.2}$$

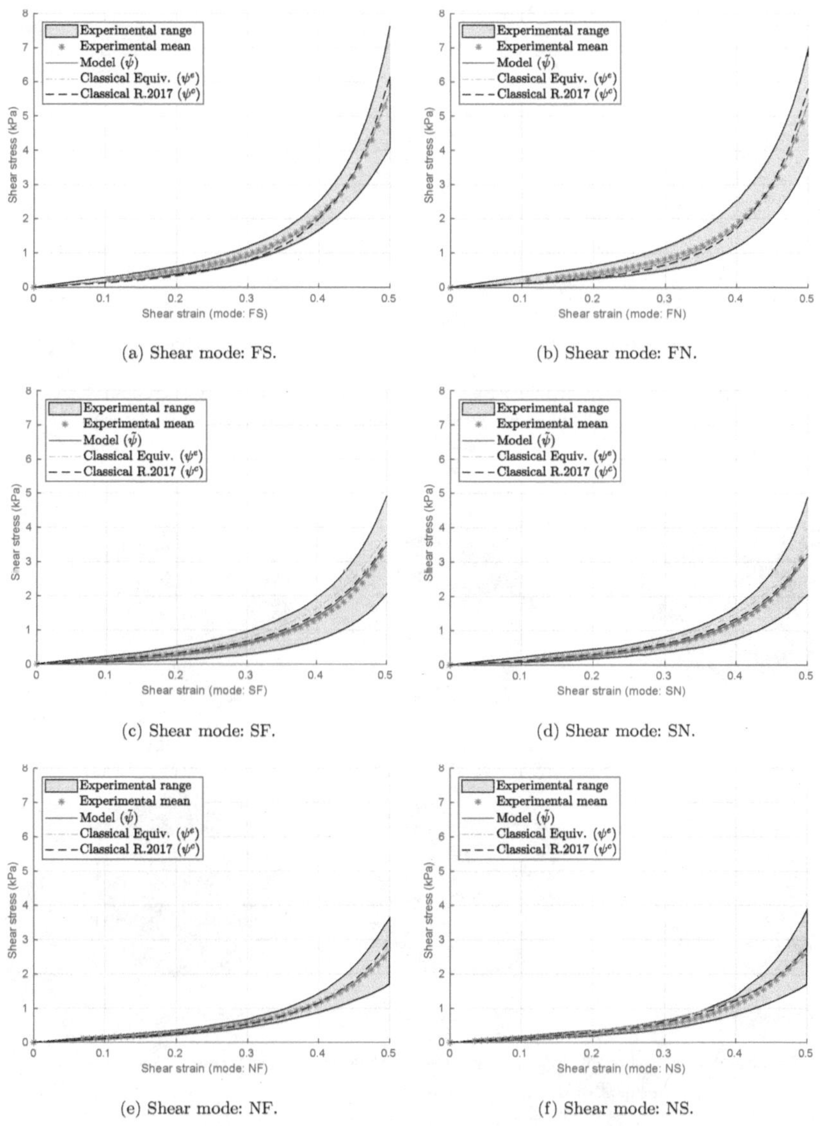


(a) Shear mode: FS.

(b) Shear mode: FN.

(c) Shear mode: SF.

(d) Shear mode: SN.

(e) Shear mode: NF.

(f) Shear mode: NS.

Fig. 6.3: The orthotropic micromorphic model ($\tilde{\psi}$) calibration graphs against triaxial shear experiment data from Sommer et al. (2015) on human cardiac tissue. The equivalent macro-scale classical model ($\psi^e$) is presented to highlight the micromorphic mixed-scale and micro-scale contributions, and the classical orthotropic model ($\psi^c$) results of Rama and Skatulla (2018) are displayed for comparison.

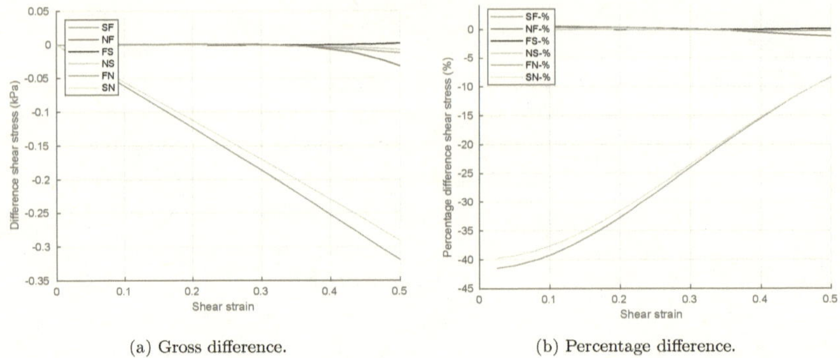


(a) Gross difference. (b) Percentage difference.

Fig. 6.4: Influence of mixed-scale and micro-scale $(\tilde{\psi}^{(1)}, \tilde{\psi}^{(2)})$ on all triaxial shear modes for the calibrated micromorphic model highlighted by difference against equivalent classical model with the same macro-scale parameters $[\sigma(\tilde{\psi}) - \sigma(\psi^e)]$.

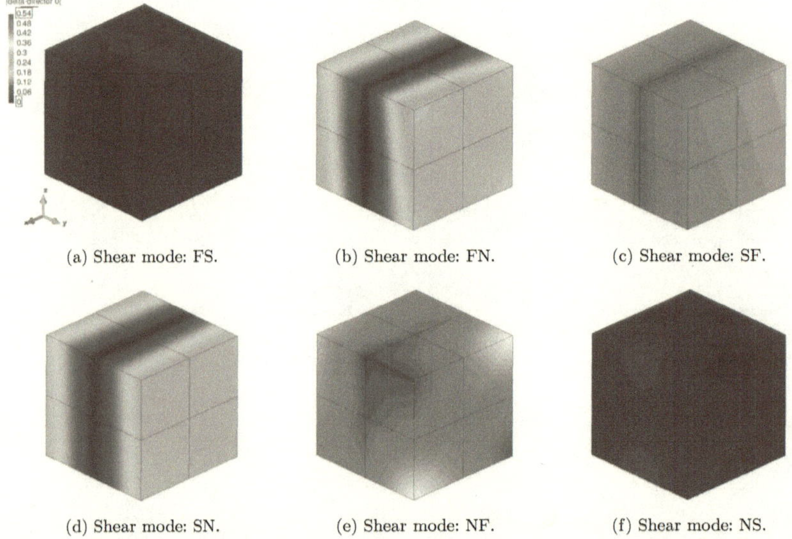

(a) Shear mode: FS. (b) Shear mode: FN. (c) Shear mode: SF.

(d) Shear mode: SN. (e) Shear mode: NF. (f) Shear mode: NS.

Fig. 6.5: The calibrated micromorphic model for the triaxial shear experiments: contour plots displaying the magnitude of displacement of the micro-directors $|\delta \mathbf{w}|$.

$$\tilde{C}^{(1)}_{j\beta} = \mathbf{F}^T \mathbf{a} = F_{rj} a_{\beta r} = \begin{bmatrix} 1 & \gamma & 0 \\ 0 & 1 & 0 \\ 0 & 0 & 1 \end{bmatrix} \begin{bmatrix} 1 + w_1 \\ w_2 \\ w_3 \end{bmatrix} = \begin{bmatrix} 1 + w_1 + \gamma w_2 \\ w_2 \\ w_3 \end{bmatrix} \tag{6.3}$$

and then the mixed-scale *Green* strain $\tilde{\mathbf{E}}^{(1)}$ with

$$\tilde{E}^{(1)}_{j\beta} = \tilde{C}^{(1)}_{j\beta} - \tilde{C}^{(1)0}_{j\beta} = \begin{bmatrix} w_1 + \gamma w_2 \\ w_2 \\ w_3 \end{bmatrix}. \tag{6.4}$$

The mixed-scale *Green* strain $\tilde{\mathbf{E}}^{(1)}$ is the only mixed-scale and micro-scale strain that can directly influence the macro-scale traction vector $\mathbf{t}^{(n)}$ in Eq. (4.57), because the micro-scale strain $\tilde{\mathbf{E}}^{(2)}$ does not feature. It can be seen that the influence of $\gamma$ is reduced by the small displacements of $w_2$. Let us compare this to a shear mode that has a more defined mixed-scale and micro-scale contribution such as the SF mode. For simple shear of $\partial u_1/\partial X_2 = \gamma$ and fibres orientated such that $\mathbf{f}^0 = \mathbf{a}^0 = \mathbf{e}_1$, we find the following mixed-scale *Green* strain:

$$\mathbf{F} = \begin{bmatrix} 1 & \gamma & 0 \\ 0 & 1 & 0 \\ 0 & 0 & 1 \end{bmatrix}, \qquad \mathbf{a} = \begin{bmatrix} 1 + w_1 \\ w_2 \\ w_3 \end{bmatrix} \tag{6.5}$$

$$\tilde{C}^{(1)}_{j\beta} = \mathbf{F}^T\mathbf{a} = F_{rj}a_{\beta r} = \begin{bmatrix} 1 & 0 & 0 \\ \gamma & 1 & 0 \\ 0 & 0 & 1 \end{bmatrix} \begin{bmatrix} 1 + w_1 \\ w_2 \\ w_3 \end{bmatrix} = \begin{bmatrix} 1 + w_1 \\ \gamma + \gamma w_1 + w_2 \\ w_3 \end{bmatrix} \tag{6.6}$$

$$\tilde{E}^{(1)}_{j\beta} = \tilde{C}^{(1)}_{j\beta} - \tilde{C}^{(1)0}_{j\beta} = \begin{bmatrix} w_1 \\ \gamma + \gamma w_1 + w_2 \\ w_3 \end{bmatrix}. \tag{6.7}$$

For the SF shear mode $\gamma$ is not diluted through multiplication with $w_i$, and therefore it can have a greater influence on $\mathbf{t}^{(n)}$ and thus the material stiffness. The shear cube models used for calibration included fibre dispersion $\mathbf{f}^0 = \mathbf{a}^0 \sim \mathbf{e}_1$, therefore the response is not as idealized as shown in Eq. (6.2)-(6.7), but is still indicative. It would be of interest to establish if the that the mixed-scale strain of the MDO micromorphic model is activated more consistently across the different shear modes, because of its differing mixed-scale strain formulation in Eq. (4.43), and this should be investigated in future work.

The mixed-scale influence was limited to a one-dimensional fibre-continuum (one micro-director) with no directional preference regarding relative shear motion between fibre and surrounding matrix. By choosing the micro-space to be three-dimensional, it would be possible to account for different relative shear motion stiffness with respect to FS and FN. Furthermore, the mixed-scale was limited to an isotropic response for this study; however, it is possible to use orthotropic constitutive law for the mixed-scale too. These additions should be utilized to improve the calibration in future studies.

## 6.2 Diastole of the left ventricle

This section describes the patient-specific ventricular geometry and corresponding boundary conditions used to model diastole of the left ventricle. A secondary calibration to a pressure-volume relationship is detailed, and results from the diastole simulation are presented.

### 6.2.1 Patient-specific ventricular geometry

At the advent of numerical modelling of the cardiac cycle, simplified geometries of the ventricles were used, such as an ellipsoid. Nowadays it is possible to model the heart more accurately using patient-specific data that better approximates the real geometry of an individual's heart. This study uses left ventricle patient-specific data processed by Hopkins (2017) who took 3D cardiac magnetic resonance (CMR) scans of the human heart provided by Cape Universities Body Imaging Centre (CUBIC), Faculty of Health Sciences UCT, Groote Schuur Hospital, Cape Town, South Africa. The data was processed into 3D models suitable for finite element simulations using the specialised segmentation software *Simpleware*. The resulting left ventricle geometry can be seen in Figure 6.6, along with the muscle fibre angles of $+66°$ for the endocardium and $-51°$ for the epicardium, as per Skatulla and Sansour (2016). The rest sarcomere lengths were prescribed as $1.91\,\mu$m on the epicardium surface and $1.78\,\mu$m on the endocardium surface [79]. The 2014 data was used in this study, which gave an end systolic volume (ESV) of 73 ml and an end diastolic volume (EDV) of 146 ml [37]. These values were used to calibrate the left ventricle model to its pressure-volume curve.

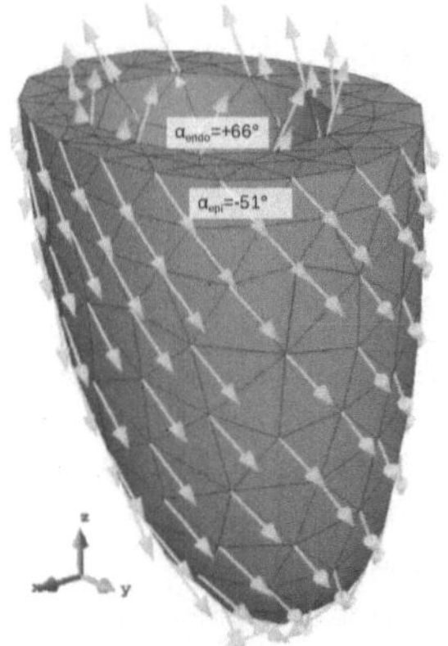


Fig. 6.6: Patient-specific left ventricle geometry for simulations from CUBIC data [37], with prescribed muscle fibre orientations at the endocardium and epicardium.

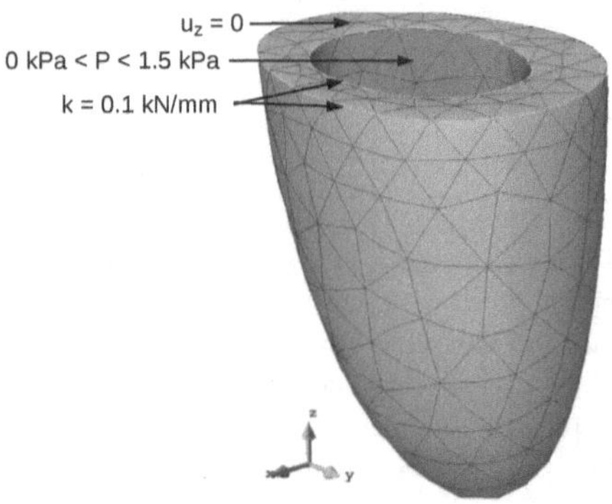

$u_z = 0$
0 kPa < P < 1.5 kPa
k = 0.1 kN/mm

Fig. 6.7: Boundary conditions applied to left ventricle model.

### 6.2.2 Boundary conditions

The choice of boundary conditions should mimic the biophysics of the left ventricle system as realistically as possible, whilst maintaining a numerically stable simulation. *Dirichlet* conditions were applied to the base to disable it from displacements in the vertical direction [1], because any structural analysis problem including the heart must be fixed at a certain location in space such that its deformation can be computed relative to it. In this sense, the rigid-body motion of heart including inertia-related effects are not reproduced but its deformation causing stress and strain can be expected to be reasonably accurate. Furthermore, the blood vessel valves at the base of the ventricle are stiff and restrict displacements [47].

$$u_z = 0 \qquad \text{on} \qquad \partial\mathcal{B}_D \tag{6.8}$$

To restrict the ventricle from rotation in the plane of the base, a circumferential elastic line force *Neumann* boundary condition of 0.1 kN/mm was applied along the epicardium and endocardium edges of the base, as this would still allow some dilation of the heart wall at the base. Another *Neumann* boundary conditions was applied to the surface of the endocardium as a cavity pressure $P$ which increased from 0 kPa to 1.5 kPa. This replicated the pressure increase as blood fills the ventricle during passive filling. The location of all the boundary conditions can be seen in Figure 6.7.

### 6.2.3 Pressure-volume curve

The calibrated material parameters listed in Table 6.1 from the triaxial experiments were applied to the left ventricle model. The triaxial shear calibration was achieved using human tissue data; however, the data was presented as mean values from a collection of samples, and thus a secondary calibration was required to better fit the model to the patient-specific heart geometry. This process was also necessary for Sack et al. (2016) who needed to adjust material parameters across species; porcine shear experiment calibrations were then re-calibrated to the pressure-volume curve of rat left ventricle data [5].

The patient-specific left ventricle had an end systolic volume (ESV) of 73 mL, and an end diastolic volume (EDV) of 146 mL for an end diastolic pressure of 1.5 kPa. It was decided that the muscle fibre contributions had already been accounted for in the shear experiment calibration, and therefore only the stiffness of the ECM would be adjusted in this pressure-volume calibration through the macro-scale stress scaling parameter $A_0$. The value of $A_0 = 0.284$ kPa taken directly from the triaxial shear experiments gave an EDV of 136 mL, which falls well within an acceptable range for a typical EDV, and therefore $A_0$ did not require much adjustment. This finding serves as good model and data validation. The successful calibration of pressure-volume is seen in Figure 6.8, and the calibrated material parameter is $A_0 = 0.194$ kPa. The results of a mesh convergence analysis are also given in Figure 6.8, and the mesh refinement accuracy had sufficiently converged at a mesh size of 1761 particles, thus this mesh size was selected for the remainder of this study.

The classical non-linear orthotropic model ($\psi^c$) of Rama and Skatulla (2018) introduced in Section 6.1.2 was again used to validate and critique the micromorphic model results in the passive filling models. Interestingly, the material parameters for $\psi^c$ shown in Table 6.1 for the triaxial shear experiments were used for the same patient-specific left ventricle model and achieved an EDV of 147.0 mL, which is extremely close to the target EDV of 146.0 mL, and therefore the material parameters were left unchanged. Similarly, the calibrated micromorphic material parameters were run in the equivalent macro-scale classical model $\psi^e$ with $A_0 = 0.194$ kPa, and the EDV achieved was 149.2 mL, and therefore the micromorphic mixed-scale and micro-scale contribution reduced the EDV by 3.2 mL.

### 6.2.4 Left ventricle models

The main objective of this research project is to assess the suitability of the micromorphic continuum model to simulate cardiac mechanics. This section contains results of simulations on the passive filling phase of the human left ventricle. The classical non-linear orthotropic model ($\psi^c$) of Rama and Skatulla (2018) introduced in Section 6.1.2 is used to validate and critique the deformations of the micromorphic model. The micromorphic model and classical model ($\psi^c$) displacement fields at the end

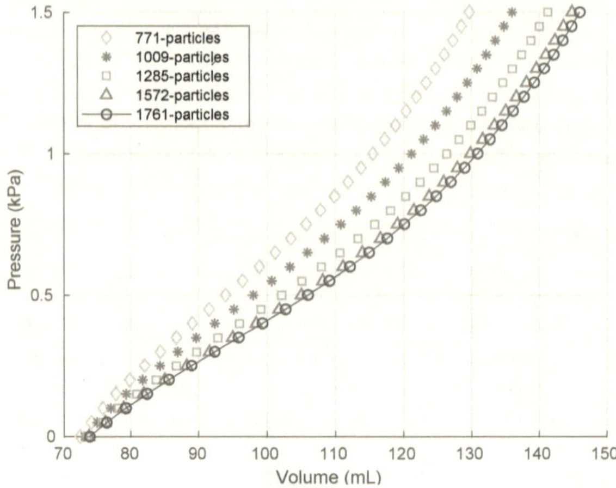


Fig. 6.8: Left ventricle pressure-volume curve during the passive filling phase for the calibrated micromorphic model with the macro-scale stress scaling parameter of $A_0 = 0.194$ kPa. Mesh convergence analysis using $A_0 = 0.194$ is shown, with the refined mesh of 1761 particles chosen for the remainder of study.

of diastolic filling are seen in Figure 6.9, and both exhibit similar patterns. The apex deforms more than the base, which is consistent with the constraining effects of the valves at the base of the heart. Also, both models deform more along the shorter diameter in the axis of the base. Subtle differences

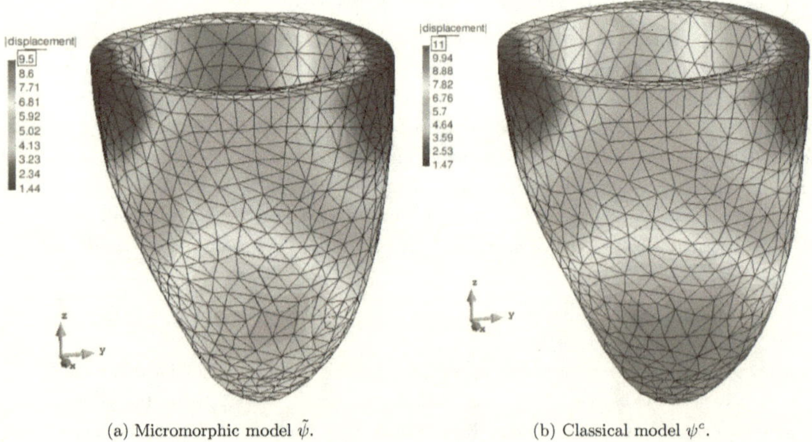


(a) Micromorphic model $\tilde{\psi}$.

(b) Classical model $\psi^c$.

Fig. 6.9: Model displacement fields for left ventricle at end of passive filling.

are evident in the fact that the classical model has larger relative displacement at the apex, whereas the micromorphic model has larger relative displacement on the short diameter towards the base.

The primary advantage of the micromorphic model for cardiac modelling is the ability to assign the muscle fibre orientation to the micromorphic micro-director. The muscle fibre orientation and stretch is of great importance to evaluate the behaviour of the ventricle. Spotnitz et al. (1974) found that the heart walls undergo larger transversal contraction during diastolic filling which has been attributed to fibre rearrangement resulting in a denser packing. The strain and stress relative to the muscle fibre is therefore displayed in Figure 6.10 and Figure 6.11, respectively. It was found in the work of Humphrey

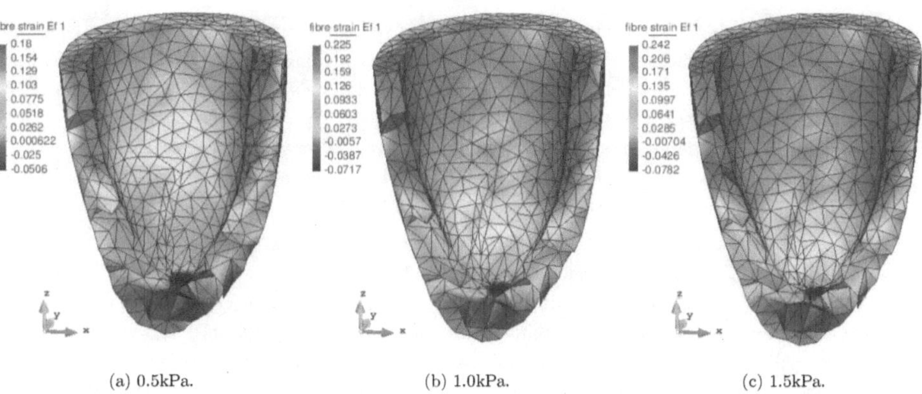


(a) 0.5kPa. (b) 1.0kPa. (c) 1.5kPa.

Fig. 6.10: Cross-section of left ventricle strain relative to muscle fibres at three intervals during passive filling using the micromorphic model.

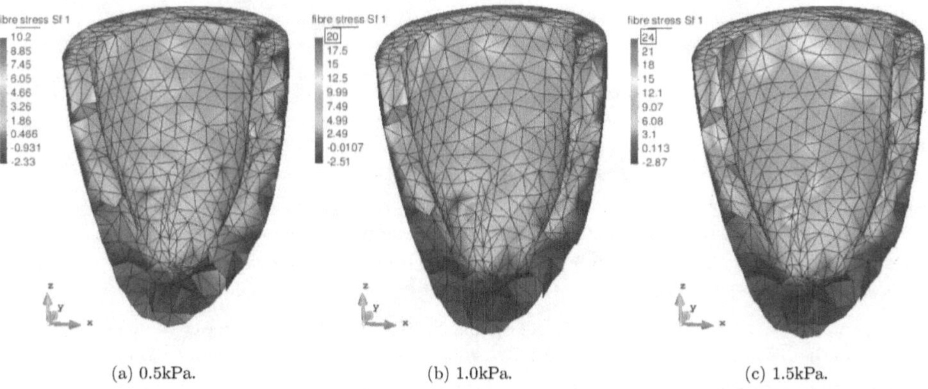


(a) 0.5kPa. (b) 1.0kPa. (c) 1.5kPa.

Fig. 6.11: Cross-section of left ventricle stress relative to muscle fibres at three intervals during passive filling using the micromorphic model.

and Yin (1989) and separately by Granzier and Irving (1995) that peak strains in the myocardium develop at the endocardium [72], which is consistent with the results by the micromorphic model.

The restriction on movement of the base of the ventricle caused by the elastic boundary condition has resulted in larger stresses developing towards the base of the heart which is to be expected. Similarly, we notice slightly larger stresses on the long diameter of the base because it did not deform as much due to the asymmetric geometry of the ventricle. The apex of the ventricle did not develop as much stress due to its larger wall thickness.

*Muscle fibre reorientation*

The ability of the micro-director to represent myocytes is crucial to the utility of the micromorphic model in cardiac mechanics. The two responses of reorientation and stretching of the micro-director during passive filling are the most suitable metrics to assess the micro-director's mimicry of the muscle fibres. However, there was a lack of clinical data to do this adequately. The clear advantage of the micromorphic model over classical models is the potential for the micro-director to move independently from the bulk material, which is referred to as non-affine motion. The non-affine motion of the micro-director is something that can be discussed in the absence of data for validation.

For classical mechanics the evolution of the undeformed myocytes $\mathbf{V}_f^{0(c)}$ to the deformed myocytes $\mathbf{V}_f^{(c)}$ is controlled by the deformation gradient, such that $\mathbf{V}_f^{(c)} = \mathbf{F}\mathbf{V}_f^{0(c)}$. This means that the myocyte deforms in the same way as the bulk material or ECM. However, the micromorphic model includes the myocytes in its degrees of freedom, and therefore the displacement $\delta\mathbf{w}_f$ of the undeformed myocytes $\mathbf{A}_f$ to the deformed myocytes $\mathbf{a}_f$ is solved intrinsically in the model and simply extracted from the global displacement vector $\mathbf{d}$. A comparison of the myocyte orientations at the end of diastolic filling for the micromorphic myocyte $\mathbf{a}_f$ and the classical myocyte $\mathbf{V}_f^{(c)}$ is seen in Figure 6.12. The final myocyte orientations are similar, which is to be expected considering that in actuality the myocytes are constrained by the ECM. However, on closer inspection there are differences between the two approximations. The classical mechanics myocyte reorientation and stretching in terms of displacement $\delta\mathbf{V}_f^{(c)}$ is calculated as

$$\delta\mathbf{V}_f^{(c)} = (\mathbf{F} - \mathbf{I})\,\mathbf{V}_f^{0(c)}. \tag{6.9}$$

The micromorphic myocyte reorientation and stretching in terms of displacements $\delta\mathbf{w}_f$ is solved directly in the model, and is merely extracted from the global displacement vector $\mathbf{d}$. To get a better understanding of the level of non-affine motion of the micro-director to the ECM, the comparison of the micro-director displacement $\delta\mathbf{w}$ against the classical displacement $\delta\mathbf{V}_f^{(c)}$ is seen in Figure 6.13. From a qualitative perspective it is clear that non-affine reorientation of the micro-director is possible with areas of significant differences in $\delta\mathbf{w}_f$ and $\delta\mathbf{V}_f^{(c)}$.

A quantitative analysis of the non-affine motions of $\delta\mathbf{w}_f$ against $\delta\mathbf{V}_f^{(c)}$ at three nodes on the epicardium of the left ventricle is presented in the graphs of Figure 6.14. The graphs show a strong trend as the micro-director displacement $\delta\mathbf{w}_f$ is almost completely opposite to that of the classically computed displacement $\delta\mathbf{V}_f^{(c)}$. This finding can perhaps be explained by the effect of the material parameters of the mixed-scale and micro-scale documented in Section 5.1.2, where micro-director displacements can be the opposite of macro-scale displacements. The finding of $\delta\mathbf{w}_f$ against $\delta\mathbf{V}_f^{(c)}$ is promising in the sense that non-affine motion of the micro-director relative to the ECM is certainly possible. However,

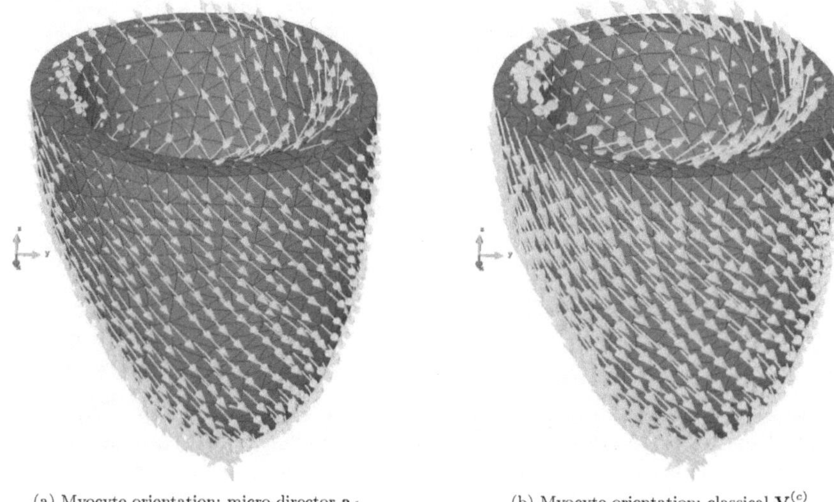

(a) Myocyte orientation: micro-director $\mathbf{a}_f$.

(b) Myocyte orientation: classical $\mathbf{V}_f^{(c)}$.

Fig. 6.12: Myocyte orientation represented by the micro director orientation $\mathbf{a}_f$ compared with classical myocyte orientation $\mathbf{V}_f^{(c)}$ at the end of diastolic filling using the micromorphic model.

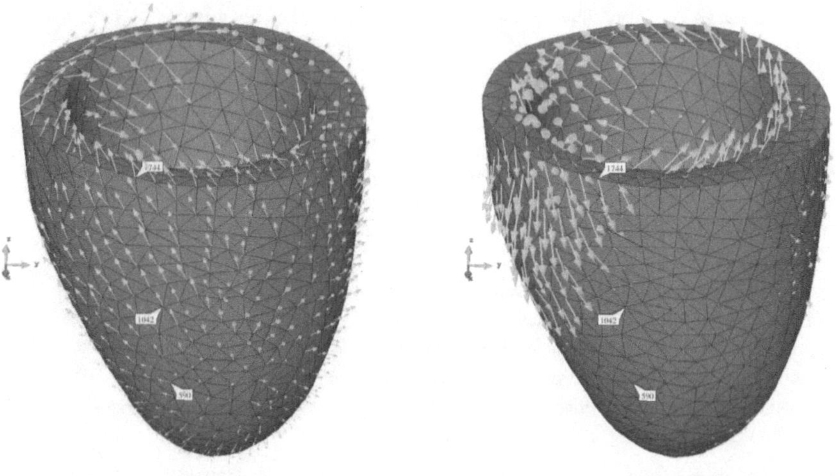

(a) Myocyte displacement: micro-director $\delta\mathbf{w}_f$.

(b) Myocyte displacement: classical $\delta\mathbf{V}_f^{(c)}$.

Fig. 6.13: Myocyte reorientation represented by the micro-director displacement $\delta\mathbf{w}_f$ and classical myocyte displacement $\delta\mathbf{V}_f^{(c)}$ at the end of diastolic filling using the micromorphic model.

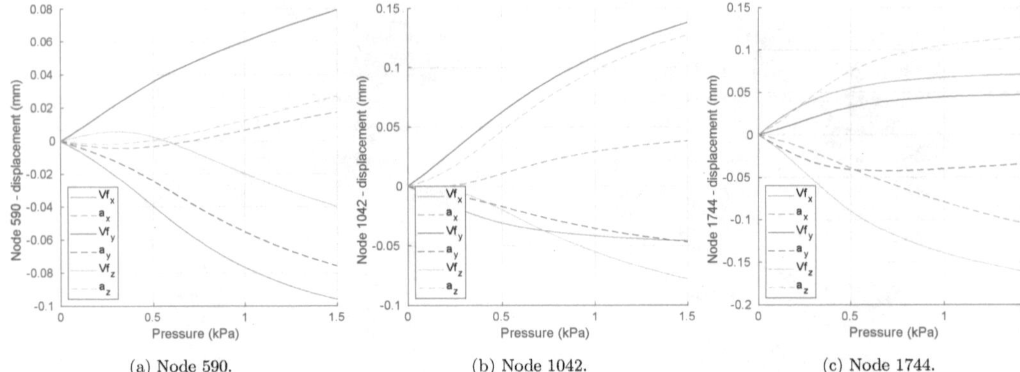


(a) Node 590. (b) Node 1042. (c) Node 1744.

Fig. 6.14: Graphs of micromorphic myocyte displacements $\delta\mathbf{w}_f$ compared with classical myocyte displacements $\delta\mathbf{V}_f^{(c)}$ to highlight non-affine myocyte motion relative to the ECM at three nodes on the epicardium of the left ventricle. Exact locations of nodes can be seen in Figure 6.13: node 1744 is at the base, node 1042 is in the middle, and node 590 is near the apex.

for the micro-director to represent myocytes accurately, a smaller difference in $\delta\mathbf{w}_f$ and $\delta\mathbf{V}_f^{(c)}$ would seem more realistic, given that the muscle fibres are constrained in the ECM. Alternatively, given that the displacement of the micro-director was almost entirely opposite that of the ECM for this specific material parameter combination, a mirrored correlation between the myocyte $\mathbf{m}_f$ and the micro-director $\mathbf{m}_f \propto -\mathbf{a}_f$ could be explored.

The assessment of the micro-director reorientation and stretching in relation to clinically observed myocyte reorientations is excluded from the scope of this work due to a lack of experimental data. Papadacci et al. (2017) were able to map myocardial fibre orientation and its reorientation over time with a temporal resolution of 10 ms using non-invasive ultrasound-based imaging technique called 3D Backscatter Tensor Imaging (BTI). This very promising technology would be of great use to better validate the reorientation of the micro-directors. The testing of further combinations of material parameters for the mixed-scale and micro-scale should be done in future work to calibrate the micro-director reorientation. However, this is likely to be an intensive process, given the abundance of material parameter combinations of the mixed-scale and micro-scale that affect the micro-director displacement. Furthermore, the fact that muscle fibres are constrained by the tissue matrix of the ECM would potentially involve some additional linkage of the macro-scale to the mixed-scale/micro-scale in the model, for example by using the penalty method.

In summary, non-affine reorientation of myocytes represented as micromorphic micro-directors relative to the ECM has been definitively achieved. However, the accuracy of the reorientation relative to clinically observed myocyte reorientation has not been assessed due to lack of data and scope limitations. Empirically, it would seem that the non-affinity of the reorientation is too pronounced, but it is hoped with more time and resources this could be improved in future work through more testing of material parameter combinations, the inclusion of the penalty method to constrain the micro-directors in the ECM, and the incorporation of micro-boundary conditions which was not investigated here.

# 7

# Conclusion

The main aim of this research was to test the suitability of the micromorphic continuum model, which was implemented by the author into the in-house software *SESKA*, to describe cardiac tissue. The testing was done in two stages: firstly, the fundamental behaviour of the micromorphic model was assessed using simple numerical examples; and secondly, cardiac tissue experiments were replicated and the passive filling phase of the left ventricle was simulated. The majority of the modelling in this study was done using Sansour's micromorphic model, which showed significant improvements in cardiac tissue simulations compared with those of a leading classical model. In addition, the author's own interpretation of the micromorphic model was developed and implemented, and it was successful in avoiding potential numerical artifacts found in Sansour's micromorphic model. The findings of the study will be summarized in this chapter, and recommendations will be made for future work using the micromorphic model in cardiac mechanics.

## 7.1 Summary of cardiac models

This study found that Sansour's generalized micromorphic model has good potential to model the heart, and improvements over classical models were achieved. The steps taken to evaluate this micromorphic model with cardiac simulations, and the subsequent findings from the cardiac modelling are summarized as follows.

Firstly, the necessary orthotropic constitutive law for modelling cardiac tissue using a micromorphic continuum was developed in Section 4.4, and it was possible to attribute separate strain energy functions for each of the kinematic scales $(\tilde{\psi}^{(0)}, \tilde{\psi}^{(1)}, \tilde{\psi}^{(2)})$. The macro-scale was given a non-linear, orthotropic constitutive law based on $\tilde{\psi}^{(0)}$, which would represent the ECM of the myocardium. The mixed-scale was given a non-linear constitutive law based on $\tilde{\psi}^{(1)}$, as it would represent the linkage, shearing and friction between the ECM and the myocytes. Finally, the micro-scale was also represented using a non-linear constitutive law based on $\tilde{\psi}^{(2)}$, as it would represent the myocytes. The ability to distinguish the strains of the components of cardiac tissue and to apply corresponding constitutive equations is a very beneficial property of the micromorphic model.

The micromorphic model was calibrated for cardiac tissue using data from triaxial shear experiments performed on human cardiac tissue by Sommer et al. (2015). The BLVM algorithm was employed to facilitate the calibration, and a range of starting material parameter combinations was tested to avoid reaching local minima. The error performance index of Eq. (6.1) for the calibrated micromorphic model was PI $= 2.44 \times 10^{-3}$, whereas the same calibration of a classical non-linear orthotropic model ($\psi^c$) done by Rama and Skatulla (2018) gave an error of PI $= 3.81 \times 10^{-3}$. Therefore, the calibration using Sansour's micromorphic model improved the performance index by 36%, and noteworthy improvements were made to the largest shear modes of FS and FN. The stress contributions from the mixed-scale and micro-scale were highlighted, and the author was able to build upon the analytical explanation offered by von Hoegen et al. (2017) to explain why certain shear modes activate the mixed-scale and micro-scale stress contributions more than other modes.

The micromorphic model was then used to model diastole of the left ventricle using patient-specific data of ventricular geometry courtesy of CUBIC, which had been processed by Hopkins (2017). The stress-scaling parameter $A_0$ was recalibrated to reach the target EDV of 146 mL. It was encouraging to note that the previously calibrated value of $A_0$ from the triaxial experiments gave an EDV of 136 mL, which was already well within in an acceptable range. The calibrated micromorphic material parameters were run in the equivalent macro-scale classical model $\psi^e$ and the EDV achieved was 149.2 mL, therefore the micromorphic mixed-scale and micro-scale contributions reduced the EDV by 3.2 mL. The micromorphic left ventricle model produced similar deformations to the classical model $\psi^c$ [66], and peak fibre strains in the myocardium developed at the endocardium of the model, which is consistent with the findings of Humphrey and Yin (1989) and separately of Granzier and Irving (1995).

The primary advantage of the micromorphic model for cardiac modelling is the ability to assign the muscle fibre orientation to the micromorphic micro-director, as the muscle fibre orientation and contracting/stretching are of great importance to evaluate the behaviour of the ventricle. The benefit of the micromorphic model over classical models is the potential for the micro-director to move independently from the bulk material, which is referred to as non-affine motion. Due to the lack of available clinical data on muscle fibre reorientation, the focus of the modelling was placed on the non-affine motion of the micro-director relative to the ECM. A quantitative analysis of the non-affine motions of the micro-director $\delta \mathbf{w}_f$ against classically computed displacements $\delta \mathbf{V}_f^{(c)}$ at three nodes on the epicardium of the left ventricle concluded that non-affine motion of the myocytes is definitely possible using the micromorphic model. However, a lack of experimental data and the scope of this project meant that the accuracy of the myocyte reorientation using the micro-directors was not determined.

## 7.2 Summary of numerical examples

The key characteristics of Sansour's micromorphic model were explored using simple model geometries, in order to make more informed decisions when applying the model to cardiac simulations. The findings of the numerical examples of Section 5 are now summarized as follows.

The numerical examples commenced with the illuminating problem of a simple tension beam under homogeneous deformation. The tension beam example was useful in showing the existence of scenarios without a unique solution, for which the micromorphic model does not solve. This phenomenon occurs for material parameter sets where the mixed-scale parameter $A_1$ and the micro-scale parameter $A_2$ are related such that $A_1 \approx -A_2$, provided there is no boundary micro-condition. The author was able to devise a novel proof for this, by breaking down the mixed-scale and micro-scale stress terms in the micro-equilibrium equation; first into the associated material parameters and strain measures, and then further into the deformation terms that constitute the strain measures. From that point, a cubic equation was derived in Eq. (5.10) relating the macro-deformation gradient $\mathbf{F}$, the micro-deformation $\mathbf{a}_\gamma$, and the material parameters $A_1, A_2$.

It was shown by the author that when $A_1 \approx -A_2$ there exist two energy minimizing micro-director deformations - an equidistant stretch or compression - that satisfy the cubic equation of Eq. (5.10). The existence of two equally suitable solutions causes the model to not solve. The author also noted the ability to calculate the micro-director deformation of a homogeneous deformation tension beam problem without running the model, but instead by simply finding the roots of Eq. (5.10), and selecting the root that is closest to $a_{\gamma 1} \to 1$. Alternatively, if the desired director displacement was known along with one of the mixed/micro parameters, it is possible to find the other corresponding calibrated mixed-scale/micro-scale parameter by substitution using Eq. (5.10), without the burden of calibrating from models using a calibration script.

The tension beam example was also used to show that the type of the micro-director deformation (stretching or contracting) under axial tension was dependent on the ratio of the material parameters $A_1 : A_2$. The author was able to attribute this behaviour to the equilibrium equations. Furthermore, it was explained in Section 5.1.2 why the micro-director can only contract if $A_1, A_2 > 0$, even though the member is under tension, and why the micro-director can make the overall material stiffer or softer in terms of the required macro-boundary traction $\hat{\mathbf{t}}^{(n)}$, depending on whether the micro-director stretches or contracts.

The fact that the micro-directors contract when the member is under tension using Sansour's model does not match what is expected of a fibrous material under axial stretching in reality - the fibres in turn would also be expected to stretch. The author thus decided that boundary micro-conditions might enforce realistic deformations. However, it was found in Section 5.2 that Sansour's micromorphic model gave spurious, non-physical micro-director deformations that were negative in sections of the member, for either prescribed positive micro-boundary force $\hat{\mathbf{q}}_\gamma^{(n)}$ or displacements $\bar{\mathbf{w}}_\gamma$. The probable cause of this issue was identified by the author and relates to Sansour's use of an analytical micro-derivative of $\tilde{\mathbf{x}}$ with respect to $\zeta^\alpha$, which results in deformation based strain measures $\mathbf{a}_\gamma$, instead of conventional strain gradient based measures $\mathbf{a}_{\gamma,i}$. The cause was described in terms of the variational formulation using Eq. (5.22), and further supported by analyzing the partitioned FEM equation system resulting in Eq. (5.28).

This motivated the author to devise an alternative micromorphic model, named the MDO model, which was set out in Section 4.2 and Section 4.3.2. It was shown in Section 5.3 that the MDO model was able to achieve micro-director stretching for the beam under tension using boundary micro-conditions, whilst maintaining all positive material parameters $A_1, A_2 > 0$ and with the desired physical result of all positive stress terms $\mathbf{S}^{(0)}, \mathbf{S}^{(1)}, \mathbf{S}^{(2)} > 0$ in the deformation direction. This scenario was not achieved with Sansour's model in this study. Furthermore, the author devised a novel proof ending in Eq. (5.40) for the critical minimum boundary micro-traction $\hat{q}_{\alpha 1}^{(\mathbf{n})} = \zeta^\alpha A_1 \left(\lambda^2 - \lambda\right)$ of Eq. (5.40) required to achieve micro-director stretching for the MDO model.

The author discovered a numerical limitation when converting the mixed-scale stress and strain tensors between Cartesian bases and natural bases, and an explanation for the problem was given in Section 5.4. The crux of the issue stems from using the curvilinear basis vectors property $\mathbf{g}_j \otimes \mathbf{g}^j = \mathbb{I}$ from Eq. (1.224) of Holzapfel (2000), and the author demonstrated why it is not valid to use this property when a one-dimensional space $\mathcal{S}(1)$ is represented using a single curvilinear basis vector that has components in three-dimensional space $\mathbb{E}(3)$. The author proposed that the bases conversion is only valid using this property when the number $(m)$ of dimensions of the micro-space $\mathcal{S}(m)$ compliments the number of dimensions of the macro-space $\mathbb{E}(m)$.

The ability of the micromorphic model to exhibit elastic strain-dependent anisotropy was highlighted in Section 5.5 with the examples of a tension beam and a perforated plate. In both scenarios it was found that under smaller strains both classical and micromorphic models exhibit significant anisotropy and produce similar deformations. However, for larger strains the classical model would continue to deform anisotropically, whereas the micromorphic micro-directors can reorientate to achieve isotropic deformations for larger strains. Strain-dependent anisotropy for classical models could only be achieved by Himpel et al. (2008) and Fausten et al. (2016) using algorithm treatment and supplementary iterative techniques, and only for dissipative reorientation not elastic reorientation achieved with the micromorphic model. The tension beam and perforated plate examples successfully replicated the results of a similar micromorphic model of von Hoegen et al. (2017), thus confirming the correct implementation of the micromorphic model in this study.

## 7.3 Recommendations and future work

The use of Sansour's generalized micromorphic model to simulate cardiac tissue has shown significant potential in this preliminary investigation. The following suggestions are made regarding recommendations for future work using the micromorphic model to describe the functioning of the heart.

The calibration of Sansour's micromorphic model to triaxial experiments was successful in reducing the error performance index compared with a leading classical model. However, considerable work is required to ensure that the contribution of the mixed-scale and micro-scale matches the contribution that the myocytes would make to the various shear modes, although current scope in this regard is limited by available clinical data. Furthermore, only one micro-director representing myocytes $\mathbf{f}$ was used, and future studies should attempt to use additional micro-directors assigned to the sheet direction $\mathbf{s}$ and the sheet-normal direction $\mathbf{n}$. The curse of dimensionality problem due to the large number of micromorphic material parameters makes the calibration process vast and would require systematic testing to converge on realistic parameter sets. The reorientation of myocytes in the triaxial experiments and the left ventricle model should be calibrated to fibre dispersion scans, such as the work of Papadacci et al. (2017) in mapping myocardial fibre reorientation using non-invasive ultrasound-based imaging technique (BTI). It is safe to say that more clinical data is required in general for cardiac mechanics, and at higher resolutions.

The finding of the micro-director deformations $\delta\mathbf{w}_f$ against the classical fibre deformations $\delta\mathbf{V}_f^{(c)}$ is promising in the sense that non-affine motion of the micro-director relative to the ECM is certainly possible. However, for the micro-director to represent myocytes accurately, a smaller difference in $\delta\mathbf{w}_f$ and $\delta\mathbf{V}_f^{(c)}$ would seem more realistic, given that the myocytes are constrained in the ECM. Alternatively, given that the displacement of the micro-director was almost entirely opposite to that of the ECM for this specific material parameter combination, a mirrored correlation between the myocyte $\mathbf{m}_f$ and the micro-director $\mathbf{a}_f$, such that $\mathbf{m}_f \propto -\mathbf{a}_f$, could be explored. Empirically, it would seem that the non-affinity of the reorientation is too pronounced; however, with more time and resources, testing of further combinations of material parameters for the mixed-scale and micro-scale, and constraining the micro-directors to the ECM using the penalty method, it is hoped that the myocyte reorientation could possibly be optimized in future work.

In regards to the numerical artifacts uncovered with the micromorphic model and the complex relationship between the mixed-scale parameter $A_1$ and the micro-scale parameter $A_2$, further investigation is certainly necessary. In particular, additional intermediate benchmarking studies on less complex materials and geometries than cardiac tissue would be useful. The author raised concerns about the ability of Sansour's generalized micromorphic model to handle boundary micro-conditions in a physically appropriate manner, and this should be investigated further. The potential benefits of the author's own MDO micromorphic model should be applied to cardiac models, and its performance should be assessed against the Sansour's micromorphic model. It is possible that the MDO model may better handle the linkage of the myocytes to the ECM, using penalty methods on the micro-scale degrees of freedom. However, the necessity of the MDO model to have boundary micro-conditions presents the challenge of realistically assigning such conditions to complex cardiac geometries, and thus further investigation is required.

In terms of modelling the cardiac cycle, this was a preliminary feasibility study, and the micromorphic model should be tested under the remaining phases of the heartbeat. In particular, the merits of applying active contraction of the myocytes through the micro-directors should be investigated. Furthermore, the use of bi-ventricular patient-specific geometries would improve the approximations of the model, and the ability to run multiple heart beats would allow for appropriate residual stresses in the ventricles, rather than starting from an unstressed state. The mechanical behaviour of the heart can be significantly altered by cardiovascular pathologies, such as cardiomyopathy, and it would be of interest to apply the micromorphic model to mimic these conditions in future work.

# A

# Supplementary Derivations

## A.1 Variants

### A.1.1 Generalized micromorphic variants

The variants of the terms making up the generalized right *Cauchy-Green* tensor $\tilde{\mathbf{C}}$ are derived here, in order to be inserted into the variational formulation of Eq. (4.50).

$$\mathbf{C}^{(0)} = (\mathbf{x}_{,k} \cdot \mathbf{x}_{,l})\ \tilde{\mathbf{G}}^k \otimes \tilde{\mathbf{G}}^l$$

$$\delta\mathbf{C}^{(0)} = (F_{rl}\,\delta u_{r,k} + F_{rk}\,\delta u_{r,l})\ \tilde{\mathbf{G}}^k \otimes \tilde{\mathbf{G}}^l \tag{A.1}$$

$$\Delta\mathbf{C}^{(0)} = (F_{rl}\,\Delta u_{r,k} + F_{rk}\,\Delta u_{r,l})\ \tilde{\mathbf{G}}^k \otimes \tilde{\mathbf{G}}^l \tag{A.2}$$

$$\Delta\delta\mathbf{C}^{(0)} = (\Delta u_{r,k}\,\delta u_{r,l} + \delta u_{r,k}\,\Delta u_{r,l})\ \tilde{\mathbf{G}}^k \otimes \tilde{\mathbf{G}}^l \tag{A.3}$$

$$\mathbf{C}^{(1)} = (\mathbf{x}_{,j} \cdot \mathbf{a}_\gamma)\ \left(\tilde{\mathbf{G}}^j \otimes \tilde{\mathbf{I}}^\gamma + \tilde{\mathbf{I}}^\gamma \otimes \tilde{\mathbf{G}}^j\right)$$

$$\begin{aligned}\delta\mathbf{C}^{(1)} &= \left(a_{\gamma r}\delta(I_{rj} + u_{r,j}) + F_{rj}\left(\frac{\partial a_\gamma}{\partial a_\phi}\right)\delta a_{\phi r}\right)\ \left(\tilde{\mathbf{G}}^j \otimes \tilde{\mathbf{I}}^\gamma + \tilde{\mathbf{I}}^\gamma \otimes \tilde{\mathbf{G}}^j\right)\\ &= (a_{\gamma r}\delta u_{r,j} + F_{rj}\delta_{\gamma\phi}\delta a_{\phi r})\ \left(\tilde{\mathbf{G}}^j \otimes \tilde{\mathbf{I}}^\gamma + \tilde{\mathbf{I}}^\gamma \otimes \tilde{\mathbf{G}}^j\right)\\ &= (a_{\gamma r}\delta u_{r,j} + F_{rj}\delta a_{\gamma r})\ \left(\tilde{\mathbf{G}}^j \otimes \tilde{\mathbf{I}}^\gamma + \tilde{\mathbf{I}}^\gamma \otimes \tilde{\mathbf{G}}^j\right)\end{aligned} \tag{A.4}$$

$$\Delta\mathbf{C}^{(1)} = (a_{\gamma s}\Delta u_{s,j} + F_{sj}\Delta a_{\gamma s})\ \left(\tilde{\mathbf{G}}^j \otimes \tilde{\mathbf{I}}^\gamma + \tilde{\mathbf{I}}^\gamma \otimes \tilde{\mathbf{G}}^j\right) \tag{A.5}$$

$$\Delta\delta\mathbf{C}^{(1)} = (\Delta a_{\gamma r}\delta u_{r,j} + \Delta u_{r,j}\delta a_{\gamma r})\ \left(\tilde{\mathbf{G}}^j \otimes \tilde{\mathbf{I}}^\gamma + \tilde{\mathbf{I}}^\gamma \otimes \tilde{\mathbf{G}}^j\right) \tag{A.6}$$

$$\mathbf{C}^{(2)} = (\mathbf{a}_\gamma \cdot \mathbf{a}_\phi)\ \tilde{\mathbf{I}}^\gamma \otimes \tilde{\mathbf{I}}^\phi$$

$$\delta\mathbf{C}^{(2)} = (\delta a_{\gamma r}a_{\phi r} + a_{\gamma r}\delta a_{\phi r})\ \tilde{\mathbf{I}}^\gamma \otimes \tilde{\mathbf{I}}^\phi \tag{A.7}$$

$$\Delta\mathbf{C}^{(2)} = (\Delta a_{\gamma s}a_{\phi s} + a_{\gamma s}\Delta a_{\phi s})\ \tilde{\mathbf{I}}^\gamma \otimes \tilde{\mathbf{I}}^\phi \tag{A.8}$$

$$\Delta\delta\mathbf{C}^{(2)} = (\delta a_{\gamma r}\Delta a_{\phi r} + \Delta a_{\gamma r}\delta a_{\phi r})\ \tilde{\mathbf{I}}^\gamma \otimes \tilde{\mathbf{I}}^\phi \tag{A.9}$$

$$\mathbf{K}^{(0)} = (\mathbf{a}_{\alpha,k} \cdot \mathbf{x}_{,l} + \mathbf{a}_{\alpha,l} \cdot \mathbf{x}_{,k})\ \tilde{\mathbf{G}}^k \otimes \tilde{\mathbf{G}}^l$$

$$\delta\mathbf{K}^{(0)} = (\delta a_{\alpha r,k}F_{rl} + a_{\alpha r,k}\delta u_{r,l} + \delta a_{\alpha r,l}F_{rk} + a_{\alpha r,l}\delta u_{r,k})\ \tilde{\mathbf{G}}^k \otimes \tilde{\mathbf{G}}^l \tag{A.10}$$

$$\Delta\mathbf{K}^{(0)} = (\Delta a_{\alpha s,k}F_{sl} + a_{\alpha s,k}\Delta u_{s,l} + \Delta a_{\alpha s,l}F_{sk} + a_{\alpha s,l}\Delta u_{s,k})\ \tilde{\mathbf{G}}^k \otimes \tilde{\mathbf{G}}^l \tag{A.11}$$

$$\Delta\delta\mathbf{K}^{(0)} = (\delta a_{\alpha r,k}\Delta u_{r,l} + \Delta a_{\alpha r,k}\delta u_{r,l} + \delta a_{\alpha r,l}\Delta u_{r,k} + \Delta a_{\alpha r,l}\delta u_{r,k})\ \tilde{\mathbf{G}}^k \otimes \tilde{\mathbf{G}}^l \tag{A.12}$$

$$\mathbf{K}^{(1)} = (\mathbf{a}_{\alpha,j} \cdot \mathbf{a}_\gamma) \left(\tilde{\mathbf{G}}^j \otimes \tilde{\mathbf{I}}^\gamma + \tilde{\mathbf{I}}^\gamma \otimes \tilde{\mathbf{G}}^j\right)$$

$$\delta\mathbf{K}^{(1)} = (\delta a_{\alpha r,j} a_{\gamma r} + a_{\alpha r,j} \delta a_{\gamma r}) \left(\tilde{\mathbf{G}}^j \otimes \tilde{\mathbf{I}}^\gamma + \tilde{\mathbf{I}}^\gamma \otimes \tilde{\mathbf{G}}^j\right) \tag{A.13}$$

$$\Delta\mathbf{K}^{(1)} = (\Delta a_{\alpha s,j} a_{\gamma s} + a_{\alpha s,j} \Delta a_{\gamma s}) \left(\tilde{\mathbf{G}}^j \otimes \tilde{\mathbf{I}}^\gamma + \tilde{\mathbf{I}}^\gamma \otimes \tilde{\mathbf{G}}^j\right) \tag{A.14}$$

$$\Delta\delta\mathbf{K}^{(1)} = (\delta a_{\alpha r,j} \Delta a_{\gamma r} + \Delta a_{\alpha r,j} \delta a_{\gamma r}) \left(\tilde{\mathbf{G}}^j \otimes \tilde{\mathbf{I}}^\gamma + \tilde{\mathbf{I}}^\gamma \otimes \tilde{\mathbf{G}}^j\right) \tag{A.15}$$

### A.1.2 MDO micromorphic variants

The variants of the terms making up the MDO right *Cauchy-Green* tensor $\check{\mathbf{C}}$ are derived here, in order to be inserted into the variational formulation of Eq. (4.60).

*Macro variants:*

$$\check{\mathbf{C}}^{(0)} = x_{r,k} x_{r,l} \left(\tilde{\mathbf{G}}^k \otimes \tilde{\mathbf{G}}^l\right)$$

$$\delta\check{\mathbf{C}}^{(0)} = (F_{rl}\, \delta u_{r,k} + F_{rk}\, \delta u_{r,l})\ \tilde{\mathbf{G}}^k \otimes \tilde{\mathbf{G}}^l \tag{A.16}$$

$$\Delta\check{\mathbf{C}}^{(0)} = (F_{sl}\, \Delta u_{s,k} + F_{sk}\, \Delta u_{s,l})\ \tilde{\mathbf{G}}^k \otimes \tilde{\mathbf{G}}^l \tag{A.17}$$

$$\Delta\delta\check{\mathbf{C}}^{(0)} = (\Delta u_{r,l}\, \delta u_{r,k} + \Delta u_{r,k}\, \delta u_{r,l})\ \tilde{\mathbf{G}}^k \otimes \tilde{\mathbf{G}}^l \tag{A.18}$$

*Mixed variants:*

$$\check{\mathbf{C}}^{(1)} = (a_{\alpha r,k} \cdot x_{r,l} + a_{\alpha r,l} \cdot x_{r,k})\ \tilde{\mathbf{G}}^k \otimes \tilde{\mathbf{G}}^l$$

$$\delta\check{\mathbf{C}}^{(1)} = (\delta a_{\alpha r,k} F_{rl} + a_{\alpha r,k} \delta u_{r,l} + \delta a_{\alpha r,l} F_{rk} + a_{\alpha r,l} \delta u_{r,k})\ \tilde{\mathbf{G}}^k \otimes \tilde{\mathbf{G}}^l \tag{A.19}$$

$$\Delta\check{\mathbf{C}}^{(1)} = (\Delta a_{\alpha s,k} F_{sl} + a_{\alpha s,k} \Delta u_{s,l} + \Delta a_{\alpha s,l} F_{sk} + a_{\alpha s,l} \Delta u_{s,k})\ \tilde{\mathbf{G}}^k \otimes \tilde{\mathbf{G}}^l \tag{A.20}$$

$$\Delta\delta\check{\mathbf{C}}^{(1)} = (\delta a_{\alpha r,k} \Delta u_{r,l} + \Delta a_{\alpha r,k} \delta u_{r,l} + \delta a_{\alpha r,l} \Delta u_{r,k} + \Delta a_{\alpha r,l} \delta u_{r,k})\ \tilde{\mathbf{G}}^k \otimes \tilde{\mathbf{G}}^l \tag{A.21}$$

*Micro variants:*

$$\check{\mathbf{C}}^{(2)} = \zeta^\alpha \zeta^\beta a_{\alpha r,m} a_{\beta r,n} \left(\tilde{\mathbf{G}}^m \otimes \tilde{\mathbf{G}}^n\right) \tag{A.22}$$

$$\delta\check{\mathbf{C}}^{(2)} = \zeta^\alpha \zeta^\beta \left[\delta a_{\alpha r,m} a_{\beta r,n} + a_{\alpha r,m} \delta a_{\beta r,n}\right] \left(\tilde{\mathbf{G}}^m \otimes \tilde{\mathbf{G}}^n\right) \tag{A.23}$$

$$\Delta\check{\mathbf{C}}^{(2)} = \zeta^\alpha \zeta^\beta \left[\Delta a_{\alpha s,m} a_{\beta s,n} + a_{\alpha s,m} \Delta a_{\beta s,n}\right] \left(\tilde{\mathbf{G}}^m \otimes \tilde{\mathbf{G}}^n\right) \tag{A.24}$$

$$\Delta\delta\check{\mathbf{C}}^{(2)} = \zeta^\alpha \zeta^\beta \left[\delta a_{\alpha r,m} \Delta a_{\beta r,n} + \Delta a_{\alpha r,m} \delta a_{\beta r,n}\right] \left(\tilde{\mathbf{G}}^m \otimes \tilde{\mathbf{G}}^n\right) \tag{A.25}$$

## A.2 Linearization

### A.2.1 Generalied micromorphic model linearization

The stiffness matrix $\Delta\delta\tilde{\Psi}(\mathbf{u}, \mathbf{w})$ is calculated as the derivative of the internal force vector $\delta\tilde{\Psi}(\mathbf{u}, \mathbf{w})$ of Eq. (4.53), and makes use of the following notation

$$\underline{\underline{\mathbb{H}}}^{(i)} = \int_S \theta \frac{\partial \tilde{\mathbf{S}}^{(i)}}{\partial \tilde{\mathbf{C}}^{(i)}}\, dS; \qquad \underline{\underline{\mathbb{H}}}^{(i)\alpha} = \int_S \theta \zeta^\alpha \frac{\partial \tilde{\mathbf{S}}^{(i)}}{\partial \tilde{\mathbf{C}}^{(i)}}\, dS; \qquad \underline{\underline{\mathbb{H}}}^{(i)\alpha\beta} = \int_S \theta \zeta^\alpha \zeta^\beta \frac{\partial \tilde{\mathbf{S}}^{(i)}}{\partial \tilde{\mathbf{C}}^{(i)}}\, dS, \tag{A.26}$$

where $\theta = 4$ for $i = 1$, else $\theta = 1/2$, because of the chosen handling of mixed-scale basis vectors double contraction, and thus we find

$$\begin{aligned}
\Delta\delta\tilde{\Psi}(\mathbf{u},\mathbf{w}) = \int_{\mathcal{B}} \Big\{ & [\mathbb{H}^{(0)pqmn} F_{sm}F_{rp} + \mathbb{H}^{(0)\alpha,pqmn} 2F_{sm}a_{\alpha r,p} + \mathbb{H}^{(0)\alpha\xi,pqmn} a_{\xi s,m}a_{\alpha r,p}]^{\delta\Delta} \Delta u_{s,n}\, \delta u_{r,q} \\
& + [\mathbb{H}^{(0)pqmn} F_{sn}F_{rp} + \mathbb{H}^{(0)\alpha,pqmn} 2F_{sn}a_{\alpha r,p} + \mathbb{H}^{(0)\alpha\xi,pqmn} a_{\xi s,n}a_{\alpha r,p}]^{\delta\Delta} \Delta u_{s,m}\, \delta u_{r,q} \\
& + [\mathbb{H}^{(1)p\gamma q\lambda} a_{\lambda s}a_{\gamma r}] \Delta u_{s,q} \delta u_{r,p} \\
& + [\mathbb{H}^{(0)\alpha,pqmn} 2F_{sm}F_{rq} + 2\mathbb{H}^{(0)\alpha\xi,pqmn} a_{\xi s,m}F_{rq}]^{\delta\Delta} \Delta u_{s,n} \delta a_{\alpha r,p} \\
& + [\mathbb{H}^{(0)\alpha,pqmn} 2F_{sm}F_{rp} + 2\mathbb{H}^{(0)\alpha\xi,pqmn} a_{\xi s,m}F_{rp}]^{\delta\Delta} \Delta u_{s,n} \delta a_{\alpha r,q} \\
& + [\mathbb{H}^{(1)\alpha,p\gamma q\lambda} a_{\lambda s}a_{\gamma r}]^{\delta\Delta} \Delta u_{s,q} \delta a_{\alpha r,p} \\
& + [\mathbb{H}^{(0)\alpha\xi,pqmn} F_{sn}F_{rq}]^{\delta\Delta} \Delta a_{\xi s,m} \delta a_{\alpha r,p} \\
& + [\mathbb{H}^{(0)\alpha\xi,pqmn} F_{sn}F_{rp}]^{\delta\Delta} \Delta a_{\xi s,m} \delta a_{\alpha r,q} \\
& + [\mathbb{H}^{(1)\alpha\xi,p\gamma q\lambda} a_{\lambda s}a_{\gamma r}] \Delta a_{\xi s,q} \delta a_{\alpha r,p} \\
& + [\mathbb{H}^{(1)p\gamma q\lambda} a_{\lambda s}F_{rp} + \mathbb{H}^{(1)\alpha,p\gamma q\lambda} a_{\lambda s}a_{\alpha r,p}]^{\delta\Delta} \Delta u_{s,q} \delta a_{\gamma r} \\
& + [\mathbb{H}^{(1)p\gamma q\lambda} F_{sq}F_{rp} + \mathbb{H}^{(1)\alpha\xi,p\gamma q\lambda} a_{\xi s,q}a_{\alpha r,p}] \Delta a_{\lambda s} \delta a_{\gamma r} \\
& + [\mathbb{H}^{(1)\alpha,p\gamma q\lambda} F_{sq}a_{\alpha r,p}]^{\delta\Delta} \Delta a_{\lambda s} \delta a_{\gamma r} \\
& + [4\,\mathbb{H}^{(2)\tau\omega\eta\phi} a_{\phi s}a_{\omega r}] \Delta a_{\eta s} \delta a_{\tau r} \\
& + [\mathbb{H}^{(1)\alpha,p\gamma q\lambda} F_{sq}a_{\gamma r} + \mathbb{H}^{(1)\alpha\xi,p\gamma q\lambda} a_{\xi s,q}a_{\gamma r}]^{\delta\Delta} \Delta a_{\lambda s} \delta a_{\alpha r,p} \Big\} dV \\
& + \int_{\mathcal{B}} \Big\{ \frac{1}{2} S^{(0)kl} [\Delta u_{r,l}\, \delta u_{r,k}]^{\delta\Delta} + M^{(0)\alpha,kl} [\Delta u_{r,l} \delta a_{\alpha r,k}]^{\delta\Delta} + \frac{1}{2} S^{(1)j\gamma} [\Delta a_{\gamma r} \delta u_{r,j}]^{\delta\Delta} \\
& + \frac{1}{2} M^{(1)\alpha,j\gamma} [\Delta a_{\gamma r} \delta a_{\alpha r,j}]^{\delta\Delta} + \frac{1}{2} S^{(2)\lambda\mu} [\Delta a_{\lambda r} \delta a_{\mu r}]^{\delta\Delta} \Big\} dV.
\end{aligned} \tag{A.27}$$

### A.2.2 MDO micromorphic model linearization

The stiffness matrix $\Delta\delta\breve{\Psi}(\mathbf{u},\mathbf{w})$ of the MDO model is calculated as the derivative of the internal force vector $\delta\breve{\Psi}(\mathbf{u},\mathbf{w})$ of Eq. (4.60), and makes use of the following notation

$$\breve{\mathbb{H}}^{(0)} = \frac{1}{2}\frac{\partial \breve{\mathbf{S}}^{(0)}}{\partial \breve{\mathbf{C}}^{(0)}}; \qquad \breve{\mathbb{H}}^{(1)\alpha\pi} = \frac{1}{2}\zeta^{\alpha}\zeta^{\pi}\frac{\partial \breve{\mathbf{S}}^{(1)}}{\partial \breve{\mathbf{C}}^{(1)}}; \qquad \breve{\mathbb{H}}^{(2)\alpha\beta\theta\varphi} = \frac{1}{2}\zeta^{\alpha}\zeta^{\beta}\zeta^{\theta}\zeta^{\varphi}\frac{\partial \breve{\mathbf{S}}^{(2)}}{\partial \breve{\mathbf{C}}^{(2)}}, \tag{A.28}$$

and hence we find

$$\begin{aligned}
\Delta\delta\breve{\Psi}(\mathbf{u},\mathbf{w}) = & \int_{\mathcal{B}} \Big\{ \breve{\mathbb{H}}^{(0)pqmn} [F_{sm}F_{rp}]^{\delta\Delta} \Delta u_{s,n} \delta u_{r,q} + \breve{\mathbb{H}}^{(0)pqmn} [F_{sn}F_{rp}]^{\delta\Delta} \Delta u_{s,m} \delta u_{r,q} \\
& + \frac{1}{2} [\breve{S}^{(0)kl}]^{\delta\Delta} \Delta u_{r,l}\, \delta u_{r,k} \Big\}\, dV \\
& + \int_{\mathcal{B}} \Big\{ \breve{\mathbb{H}}^{(1)\alpha\pi,ptql} [a_{\alpha s,q}F_{rt}]^{\delta\Delta} \Delta u_{s,l} \delta a_{\pi r,p} + \breve{\mathbb{H}}^{(1)\alpha\pi,ptql} [a_{\alpha s,l}F_{rt}]^{\delta\Delta} \Delta u_{s,q} \delta a_{\pi r,p} \\
& + \breve{\mathbb{H}}^{(1)\alpha\pi,ptql} [a_{\alpha s,q}F_{rp}]^{\delta\Delta} \Delta u_{s,l} \delta a_{\pi r,t} + \breve{\mathbb{H}}^{(1)\alpha\pi,ptql} [a_{\alpha s,l}F_{rp}]^{\delta\Delta} \Delta u_{s,q} \delta a_{\pi r,t} \\
& + \frac{1}{2} [\breve{S}^{(1)\alpha,jl}]^{\delta\Delta} \Delta u_{r,l} \delta a_{\alpha r,j} + \frac{1}{2} [\breve{S}^{(1)\alpha,jl}]^{\delta\Delta} \Delta u_{r,j} \delta a_{\alpha r,l} \Big\}\, dV \\
& + \int_{\mathcal{B}} \Big\{ \breve{\mathbb{H}}^{(2)\alpha\beta\theta\varphi,pqmn} [a_{\beta s,n}a_{\varphi r,q}]^{\delta\Delta} \Delta a_{\alpha s,m} \delta a_{\theta r,p} \\
& + \breve{\mathbb{H}}^{(2)\alpha\beta\theta\varphi,pqmn} [a_{\beta s,n}a_{\theta r,p}]^{\delta\Delta} \Delta a_{\alpha s,m} \delta a_{\varphi r,q} \\
& + \frac{1}{2} [\breve{S}^{(2)\alpha\beta,mn}]^{\delta\Delta} \Delta a_{\alpha r,m} \delta a_{\beta r,n} \Big\}\, dV.
\end{aligned} \tag{A.29}$$

# B

# SESKA

The in-house C++ software *SESKA* has been developed by Assoc. Prof. Sebastian Skatulla and his students for over a decade. The software solves continuum mechanics problems using the element free Galerkin method (EFG) and the Finite Element Method (FEM) based approximations. All necessary calculations are contained in the code with some assistance of several external code libraries. *SESKA* is advantageous as it has been parallelized and thus simulations can be solved over multiple processors (CPU's) through the *Message Passing Interface* (MPI) standard library. As such, it can be used on desktop computers as well as on high-performance computer clusters to allow for higher-resolution modelling.

Non-linear problems are solved using a Newton Raphson scheme, while shape-functions and derivatives are calculated using the MLS method. The commercial software *GiD* is used for pre/post-processing, such as assigning boundary conditions to the geometry or visualizing solutions. The main external libraries employed by *SESKA* follow:

- **Portable, Extensible Toolkit for Scientific Computation (PETSc)** is used for solving partial differential equations (PDE's) for massive data problems using MPI. Numerical stability is improved through the use of preconditioners. PETSc has efficient routines to deal with sparse matrices common in computational mechanics problems.
- **ParMetis** is a parallelised library that produces efficient mesh partitioning and sparse matrices for rapid solving.
- **Linear Algebra Package (LAPACK)** is fortran code for numerical linear algebra, such as linear equation solving and eigenvalue problems.
- **Basic Linear Algebra Subprogram (BLAS)** executes common linear algebra operations, such as vector/matrix operations.

# C

# Ethics Form

Application for Approval of Ethics in Research (EiR) Projects
Faculty of Engineering and the Built Environment, University of Cape Town

## APPLICATION FORM

**Please Note:**

| APPLICANT'S DETAILS | | |
|---|---|---|
| Name of principal researcher, student or external applicant | | Devin Dollery |
| Department | | Civil Engineering |
| Preferred email address of applicant | | dlldev001@myuct.ac.za |
| If a Student | Your Degree e.g., MSc, PhD, etc. | MSc |
| | Name of Supervisor (if supervised) | Dr Sebastian Skatulla |
| If this is a researchcontract, indicate the source of funding/sponsorship | | NRF / Departmental |
| Project Title | | Development of a Micro-Structure-Motivated Material Model (Micromorphic Continuum) for Myocardial Tissue. |

- 
- 
- 
- 
- 
- 

| SIGNED BY | Full name | Signature | Date |
|---|---|---|---|
| **Principal Researcher/ Student/External applicant** | Devin Dollery | | |

| APPLICATION APPROVED BY | Full name | Signature | Date |
|---|---|---|---|
| **Supervisor** (where applicable) | Dr Sebastian Skatulla | | 2/11/16 |
| **HOD (or delegated nominee)** Final authority for all applicants who have answered NO to all questions in Section1, and for all Undergraduateresearch (including Honours) | | | |
| **Chair : Faculty EIR Committee** For applicants other than undergraduate students who have answered YES to any of the above questions | | | |

Page 1 of 1

Fig. C.1: Ethics form.

# References


[1] J. Aguado-Sierra, A. Krishnamurthy, C. Villongco, J. Chuang, E. Howard, M. J. Gonzales, J. Omens, D. E. Krummen, S. Narayan, R. C. P. Kerckhoffs, and A. D. McCulloch. Patient-specific modeling of dyssynchronous heart failure: A case study. *Progress in Biophysics and Molecular Biology*, 107(1):147–155, 2011. ISSN 0079-6107. doi: https://doi.org/10.1016/j.pbiomolbio.2011.06.014.

[2] M. A. Bessa, R. Bostanabad, Z. Liu, A. Hu, D. W. Apley, C. Brinson, W. Chen, and W. K. Liu. A framework for data-driven analysis of materials under uncertainty: Countering the curse of dimensionality. *Computer Methods in Applied Mechanics and Engineering*, 320:633–667, 2017. ISSN 00457825. doi: 10.1016/j.cma.2017.03.037.

[3] P. H. M. Bovendeerd, J. Rijcken, D. H. Van Campen, A. J. G. Schoofs, K. Nicolay, and T. Arts. Optimization of Left Ventricular Muscle Fiber Orientation BT - IUTAM Symposium on Synthesis in Bio Solid Mechanics. pages 285–296, Dordrecht, 2002. Springer Netherlands. ISBN 978-0-306-46939-8.

[4] C. J. Chuong and Y. C. Fung. Three-Dimensional Stress Distribution in Arteries. *Journal of Biomechanical Engineering*, 105(3):268, 1983. ISSN 0148-0731. doi: 10.1115/1.3138417.

[5] O. H. Cingolani, X. P. Yang, M. A. Cavasin, and O. A. Carretero. Increased systolic performance with diastolic dysfunction in adult spontaneously hypertensive rats. *Hypertension*, 41(2):249–254, 2003. ISSN 0194911X. doi: 10.1161/01.HYP.0000052832.96564.0B.

[6] S. Cooreman, D. Lecompte, H. Sol, J. Vantomme, and D. Debruyne. Elasto-plastic material parameter identification by inverse methods: Calculation of the sensitivity matrix. *International Journal of Solids and Structures*, 44(13):4329–4341, 2007. ISSN 00207683. doi: 10.1016/j.ijsolstr.2006.11.024.

[7] E. Cosserat and F. Cosserat. *Theorie des corps deformables*. A. Hermann et fils, 1909.

[8] K. D. Costa, J. W. Holmes, and A. D. McCulloch. Modelling Cardiac Mechanical Properties in Three Dimensions. *Philosophical Transactions: Mathematical, Physical and Engineering Sciences*, 359(1783):1233–1250, 2001. ISSN 1364503X. URL `http://www.jstor.org.ezproxy.uct.ac.za/stable/3066567`.

[9] R. Dal-Re. Worldwide Behavioral Research on Major Global Causes of Mortality. *Health Education & Behavior*, 38(5):433–440, 2011. ISSN 1090-1981. doi: 10.1177/1090198111402197.

[10] R. De-Carvalho, R. A. Valente, and A. Andrade-Campos. Optimization strategies for non-linear material parameters identification in metal forming problems. *Computers and Structures*, 89(1-2):246–255, 2011. ISSN 00457949. doi: 10.1016/j.compstruc.2010.10.002.

[11] P. P. De Tombe and H. E. Ter Keurs. The velocity of cardiac sarcomere shortening: Mechanisms and implications. *Journal of Muscle Research and Cell Motility*, 33(6):431–437, 2012. ISSN 01424319. doi: 10.1007/s10974-012-9310-0.

[12] S. Dokos, B. H. Smaill, A. a. Young, and I. J. LeGrice. Shear properties of passive ventricular myocardium. *American journal of physiology. Heart and circulatory physiology*, 283(6):H2650–H2659, 2002. ISSN 0363-6135. doi: 10.1152/ajpheart.00111.2002.

[13] A. Elías-Zúñiga, K. Baylon, I. Ferrer, L. Serenó, M. L. Garcia-Romeu, I. Bagudanch, J. Grabalosa, T. Pérez-Recio, O. Martinez-Romero, W. Ortega, and L. Elizalde. On the rule of mixtures for predicting stress-softening and residual strain effects in biological tissues and biocompatible materials. *Materials*, 7, 12 2013. doi: 10.3390/ma7010441.

[14] J. Ericksen and C. Truesdell. Exact theory of stress and strain in rods and shells. *Archive for Rational Mechanics and Analysis*, 1(1):295–323, 1957. ISSN 0003-9527. doi: 10.1007/BF00298012.

[15] A. Eringen and E. Suhubi. Nonlinear theory of simple micro-elastic solids - I. *International In*, 2(2):189–203, 1964. ISSN 00207225. doi: 10.1016/0020-7225(64)90004-7.

[16] A. C. Eringen. Mechanics of micromorphic materials. In *11th international congress of applied mechanics*, pages 131–138. 1966. ISBN 978-3-662-30259-0. doi: 10.1007/978-3-662-29364-5_12.

[17] A. C. Eringen. Linear Theory of Micropolar Elasticity. *Journal of Mathematics and Mechanics*, 15 (6):909–923, 1966. ISSN 00959057, 19435274. URL `http://www.jstor.org/stable/24901442`.

[18] A. C. Eringen. *Microcontinuum Field Theories - I: Foundations and Solids*. Springer, New York, 1999.

[19] S. Fausten, D. Balzani, and J. Schröder. An algorithmic scheme for the automated calculation of fiber orientations in arterial walls. *Computational Mechanics*, 58(5):861–878, 2016. ISSN 1432-0924. doi: 10.1007/s00466-016-1321-z.

[20] J. Fish. *Finite Elements A First Course in Finite Elements*. Wiley, 2007. ISBN 9780470035801.

[21] G. M. Fomovsky, S. Thomopoulos, and J. W. Holmes. Contribution of extracellular matrix to the mechanical properties of the heart. *Journal of Molecular and Cellular Cardiology*, 48(3):490–496, 2010. ISSN 00222828. doi: 10.1016/j.yjmcc.2009.08.003.

[22] Y. C. Fung, K. Fronek, and P. Patitucci. Pseudoelasticity of arteries and the choice of its mathematical expression. *American Journal of Physiology-Heart and Circulatory Physiology*, 237(5):H620–H631, nov 1979. ISSN 0363-6135. doi: 10.1152/ajpheart.1979.237.5.H620.

[23] M. G. D. Geers, E. W. C. Coenen, and V. G. Kouznetsova. Multi-scale computational homogenization of structured thin sheets. *Modelling and Simulation in Materials Science and Engineering*, 15(4), 2007. ISSN 09650393. doi: 10.1088/0965-0393/15/4/S06.

[24] H. Ghaemi, K. Behdinan, and A. D. Spence. In vitro technique in estimation of passive mechanical properties of bovine heart. Part II. Constitutive relation and finite element analysis. *Medical Engineering and Physics*, 31(1):83–91, 2009. doi: 10.1016/j.medengphy.2008.04.009.

[25] S. H. Gilbert, A. P. Benson, P. Li, and A. V. Holden. Regional localisation of left ventricular sheet structure: integration with current models of cardiac fibre, sheet and band structure. *European Journal of Cardio-thoracic Surgery*, 32(2):231–249, 2007. doi: 10.1016/j.ejcts.2007.03.032.

[26] H. L. Granzier and T. C. Irving. Passive tension in cardiac muscle: contribution of collagen, titin, microtubules, and intermediate filaments. *Biophysical Journal*, 68(3):1027–1044, 1995. ISSN 00063495. doi: 10.1016/S0006-3495(95)80278-X.

[27] R. A. Greenbaum, S. Y. Ho, D. G. Gibson, A. E. Becker, and R. H. Anderson. Left ventricular fibre architecture in man. *British Heart Journal*, 45(3):248, 1981. doi: 10.1136/hrt.45.3.248.

[28] K. B. Gupta, M. B. Ratcliffe, M. A. Fallert, L. H. Edmunds, and D. K. Bogen. Changes in passive mechanical stiffness of myocardial tissue with aneurysm formation. *Circulation*, 89(5):2315–2326, 1994. ISSN 00097322. doi: 10.1161/01.CIR.89.5.2315.

[29] A. C. Guyton. *Textbook of medical physiology*. Elsevier Saunders, Philadelphia, 11th ed. edition, 2006. ISBN 0721602401.

[30] W. Hare, J. Nutini, and S. Tesfamariam. A survey of non-gradient optimization methods in structural engineering. *Advances in Engineering Software*, 59:19–28, 2013. ISSN 09659978. doi: 10.1016/j.advengsoft.2013.03.001.

[31] I. Hariton, G. DeBotton, T. C. Gasser, and G. A. Holzapfel. Stress-driven collagen fiber re-modeling in arterial walls. *Journal of Biomechanics*, 39:S317, 2006. ISSN 0021-9290. doi: https://doi.org/10.1016/S0021-9290(06)84245-4.

[32] Health Appointments. Basic cardiac structure, 2018. URL `https://healtheappointments.com/chapter-1-basic-cardiac-structure`.

[33] G. Himpel, A. Menzel, E. Kuhl, and P. Steinmann. Time-dependent fibre reorientation of transversely isotropic continua - Finite element formulation and consistent linearization. *International Journal for Numerical Methods in Engineering*, 73(10):1413–1433, 2008. doi: 10.1002/nme.2124.

[34] G. Holzapfel. *Nonlinear solid mechanics: A continuum approach for engineering*, volume First Edit. 2000. ISBN 0471823198. doi: 10.1023/A:1020843529530.

[35] G. A. Holzapfel and R. W. Ogden. Constitutive modelling of passive myocardium: a structurally based framework for material characterization. *Philosophical Transactions of the Royal Society A: Mathematical, Physical and Engineering Sciences*, 367(1902):3445 LP – 3475, sep 2009. URL `http://rsta.royalsocietypublishing.org/content/367/1902/3445.abstract`.

[36] G. A. Holzapfel, T. C. Gasser, and R. W. Ogden. A new constitutive framework for arterial wall mechanics and a comparative study of material models. *Journal of Elasticity*, 61(1-3):1–48, 2000. ISSN 03743535. doi: 10.1023/A:1010835316564.

[37] G. Hopkins. *Growth, modelling and remodelling of cardiac tissue: a multiphase approach*. Masters book, University of Cape Town, 2017.

[38] G. Hopkins, S. Skatulla, L. Moj, T. Ricken, N. Ntusi, and E. Meintjes. A biphasic model for full cycle simulation of the human heart aimed at rheumatic heart disease. *Computers and Structures*, 2018. ISSN 0045-7949. doi: 10.1016/j.compstruc.2018.02.012.

[39] D. Humphrey and C. P. Yin. Constitutive Relations and Finite Deformations of Passive Cardiac Tissue II: Stress Analysis in the Left Ventricle. *Circulation Research*, 65(3):805–817, 1989. ISSN 0009-7330. doi: 10.1161/01.RES.65.3.805.

[40] J. D. Humphrey. Mechanics of the Arterial Wall: Review and Directions. *Critical reviews in biomedical engineering*, 23:1–162, feb 1995.

[41] J. D. Humphrey and F. C. Yin. A new constitutive formulation for characterizing the mechanical behavior of soft tissues. *Biophysical Journal*, 52(4):563–570, 1987. doi: 10.1016/S0006-3495(87)83245-9.

[42] J. R. Hussan, M. L. Trew, and P. J. Hunter. A Mean-field Model of Ventricular Muscle Tissue. *Journal of Biomechanical Engineering*, 134(7):071003, 2012. doi: 10.1115/1.4006850.

[43] Y. Kanzaki, F. Terasaki, M. Okabe, S. Fujita, T. Katashima, K. Otsuka, and N. Ishizaka. Three-dimensional architecture of cardiomyocytes and connective tissue in human heart revealed by scanning electron microscopy. *Circulation*, 122(19):1973–1974, 2010. ISSN 00097322. doi: 10.1161/CIRCULATIONAHA.110.979815.

[44] A. M. Katz. *Physiology of the heart.* Wolters Kluwer Health/Lippincott Williams & Wilkins Health, Philadelphia, PA, 5th ed. edition, 2011. ISBN 9781608311712.

[45] J. C. Kentish, H. E. Ter Keurs, L. Ricciardi, J. J. Bucx, and M. I. Noble. Comparison between the sarcomere length-force relations of intact and skinned trabeculae from rat right ventricle. Influence of calcium concentrations on these relations. *Circulation Research*, 58(6):755–768, 1986. ISSN 00097330. doi: 10.1161/01.RES.58.6.755.

[46] R. C. Kerckhoffs, P. H. Bovendeerd, J. C. Kotte, F. W. Prinzen, K. Smits, and T. Arts. Homogeneity of cardiac contraction despite physiological asynchrony of depolarization: A model study. *Annals of Biomedical Engineering*, 31(5):536–547, 2003. ISSN 00906964. doi: 10.1114/1.1566447.

[47] G. Krishnamurthy, D. Ennis, A. Itoh, W. Bothe, J. Swanson, M. Karlsson, E. Kuhl, D. Miller, and N. Ingels. Material properties of the ovine mitral valve anterior leaflet in vivo from inverse finite element analysis. *American Journal of Physiology*, 295(3):H1141, 2008. ISSN 03636135. doi: 10.1152/ajpheart.00284.2008.

[48] W. M. Lai, D. Rubin, and E. Krempl. *Introduction to Continuum Mechanics (Fourth Edition).* 2010. ISBN 978-0-75-068560-3.

[49] R. Le Riche and F. Guyon. Least Squares Parameter Estimation and the Levenberg-Marquardt Algorithm : Deterministic Analysis, Sensitivities and Numerical Experiments. Technical report, Technical Report no. 041/99, Ecole des Mines de Saint-Étienne, Saint-Étienne, France, 2000.

[50] J. D. Lee and X. Wang. Generalized Micromorphic solids and fluids. *International Journal of Engineering Science*, 49(12):1378–1387, 2011. ISSN 00207225. doi: 10.1016/j.ijengsci.2011.04.001.

[51] D. Legner, S. Skatulla, J. Mbewu, R. R. Rama, B. D. Reddy, C. Sansour, N. H. Davies, and T. Franz. Studying the influence of hydrogel injections into the infarcted left ventricle using the element-free Galerkin method. *International Journal for Numerical Methods in Biomedical Engineering*, 30(3):416–429, 2014. ISSN 20407947. doi: 10.1002/cnm.2610.

[52] I. J. LeGrice, B. H. Smaill, L. Z. Chai, S. G. Edgar, J. B. Gavin, and P. J. Hunter. Laminar structure of the heart: ventricular myocyte arrangement and connective tissue architecture in the dog. *Am J Physiol*, 269(2 Pt 2):H571–82, 1995. ISSN 0002-9513. doi: 10.1161/HC1002.105231.

[53] K. Levenberg. A method for the solution of certain non-linear problems in least squares. *Quarterly of Applied Mathematics*, 2(2):164–168, 1944. ISSN 0033-569X. doi: 10.1090/qam/10666.

[54] X. Li and H. S. Yu. Macro–micro relations in granular mechanics. *International Journal of Solids and Structures*, 46(25):4331–4341, 2009. ISSN 0020-7683. doi: https://doi.org/10.1016/j.ijsolstr.2009.08.018.

[55] R. Lozano, M. Naghavi, and K. Foreman. Global and regional mortality from 235 causes of death for 20 age groups in 1990 and 2010: a systematic analysis for the Global Burden of Disease Study 2010. *The Lancet*, 380(9859):2095–2128, 2012. doi: 10.1016/S0140-6736(12)61728-0.

[56] G. Macgowan, E. Shapiro, H. Azhari, and C. Siu. Noninvasive measurement of shortening in the fiber and cross-fiber directions in the normal human left ventricle and in idiopathic dilated cardiomyopathy. *Circulation*, 96(2):535–541, 1997. ISSN 00097322. doi: 10.1161/01.CIR.96.2.535.

[57] D. Marquardt. An Algorithm for Least-Squares Estimation of Nonlinear Parameters. *Journal of the Society for Industrial and Applied Mathematics*, 11(2):431–441, jun 1963. ISSN 0368-4245. doi: 10.1137/0111030.

[58] J. R. Martina, P. H. M. Bovendeerd, N. de Jonge, B. A. J. M. de Mol, J. R. Lahpor, and M. C. M. Rutten. Simulation of changes in myocardial tissue properties during left ventricular

assistance with a rotary blood pump. *Artificial Organs*, 37(6):531–540, 2013. ISSN 0160564X. doi: 10.1111/j.1525-1594.2012.01548.x.

[59] R. D. Mindlin. Micro-structure in linear elasticity. *Archive for Rational Mechanics and Analysis*, 16(1):51–78, 1964. ISSN 1432-0673. doi: 10.1007/BF00248490.

[60] P. M. Nielsen, I. J. Le Grice, B. H. Smaill, and P. J. Hunter. Mathematical model of geometry and fibrous structure of the heart. *The American journal of physiology*, 260(4 Pt 2):H1365–78, 1991. ISSN 0002-9513.

[61] E. Onate, F. J. Bellomo, V. Monteiro, S. Oller, and L. G. Nallim. *Characterization of Mechanical Properties of Biological Tissue: Application to the FEM Analysis of the Urinary Bladder.* John Wiley and Sons, Ltd, 2013. ISBN 9781118402955. doi: 10.1002/9781118402955.ch15.

[62] L. H. Opie. *The heart : physiology and metabolism.* Raven, New York, 2nd ed edition. ISBN 0881677511.

[63] C. Papadacci, V. Finel, J. Provost, O. Villemain, P. Bruneval, J.-l. Gennisson, M. Tanter, M. Fink, and M. Pernot. Imaging the dynamics of cardiac fiber orientation in vivo using 3D Ultrasound Backscatter Tensor Imaging. *Scientific Reports*, (November 2016):1–9, 2017. ISSN 2045-2322. doi: 10.1038/s41598-017-00946-7.

[64] S. Pranesh and D. Ghosh. Addressing the curse of dimensionality in SSFEM using the dependence of eigenvalues in KL expansion on domain size. *Computer Methods in Applied Mechanics and Engineering*, 311:457–475, 2016. ISSN 0045-7825. doi: https://doi.org/10.1016/j.cma.2016.08.023.

[65] R. R. Rama. *Proper orthogonal decomposition with interpolation-based real-time modelling of the heart.* PhD book, University of Cape Town, 2017.

[66] R. R. Rama and S. Skatulla. Towards real-time cardiac mechanics modelling with patient-specific heart anatomies. *Comput. Methods Appl. Mech. Eng.*, 328:47–74, 2018. ISSN 0045-7825. doi: 10.1016/j.cma.2017.08.015.

[67] R. R. Rama, S. Skatulla, and C. Sansour. Real-time modelling of diastolic filling of the heart using the proper orthogonal decomposition with interpolation. *International Journal of Solids and Structures*, 96:409–422, 2016. ISSN 0020-7683. doi: 10.1016/j.ijsolstr.2016.04.003.

[68] Research Cardio. Layers of cardiac tissue, 2018. URL `http://www.cardio-research.com/basic-anatomy-of-the-human-heart`.

[69] J. Rijcken, P. H. Bovendeerd, A. J. Schoofs, D. H. van Campen, and T. Arts. Optimization of Cardiac Fibre Orientation for Homogeneous Fibre Strain During Ejection. *Annual Biomedical Engineering*, 27(10):289–297, oct 1999. ISSN 0021-9290. doi: 10.1016/S0021-9290(97)00064-X.

[70] D. E. Roberts, L. T. Hersh, and A. M. Scher. Influence of Cardiac Fiber Orientation on Wavefront Voltage, Conduction Velocity, and Tissue Resistivity in the Dog. *Circulation Research*, 44(5):701–711, 1979. ISSN 0009-7330. doi: 10.1161/01.RES.44.5.701.

[71] D. Rohmer, A. Sitek, and G. T. Gullberg. Reconstruction and Visualization of Fiber and Laminar Structure in the Normal Human Heart from Ex Vivo DTMRI Data. *Investigative Radiology*, 42 (11):777–789, 2007.

[72] K. L. Sack, S. Skatulla, and C. Sansour. Biological tissue mechanics with fibres modelled as one-dimensional Cosserat continua. Applications to cardiac tissue. *International Journal of Solids and Structures*, 81:84–94, 2016. ISSN 0020-7683. doi: https://doi.org/10.1016/j.ijsolstr.2015.11.009.

[73] C. Sansour. A unified concept of elastic-viscoplastic Cosserat and micromorphic continua. *Journal de Physique IV Proceeding*, 8:341–348, 1998. ISSN 11554339.

[74] C. Sansour and S. Skatulla. A strain gradient generalized continuum approach for modelling elastic scale effects. *Computer Methods in Applied Mechanics and Engineering*, 198(15-16):1401–1412, 2009. ISSN 00457825. doi: 10.1016/j.cma.2008.12.031.

[75] C. Sansour, S. Skatulla, and H. Zbib. A formulation for the micromorphic continuum at finite inelastic strains. *International Journal of Solids and Structures*, 47(11-12):1546–1554, 2010. ISSN 00207683. doi: 10.1016/j.ijsolstr.2010.02.017.

[76] J. Schröder. A numerical two-scale homogenization scheme: the FE2-method. In J. Schröder and K. Hackl, editors, *Plasticity and Beyond: Microstructures, Crystal-Plasticity and Phase Transitions*, pages 1–64. Springer Vienna, Vienna, 2014. doi: 10.1007/978-3-7091-1625-8_1.

[77] M. S. Sirry, J. R. Butler, S. S. Patnaik, B. Brazile, R. Bertucci, A. Claude, R. McLaughlin, N. H. Davies, J. Liao, and T. Franz. Characterisation of the mechanical properties of infarcted myocardium in the rat under biaxial tension and uniaxial compression. *Journal of the Mechanical Behavior of Biomedical Materials*, 63:252–264, 2016. doi: 10.1016/j.jmbbm.2016.06.029.

[78] S. Skatulla. *PhD book: Computational Aspects of Generalized Continua based on Moving Least Square Approximations.* PhD book, University of Adelaide, 2006.

[79] S. Skatulla and C. Sansour. On a path-following method for non-linear solid mechanics with applications to structural and cardiac mechanics subject to arbitrary loading scenarios. *International Journal of Solids and Structures*, 96:181–191, 2016. ISSN 0020-7683. doi: 10.1016/j.ijsolstr.2016.06.009.

[80] G. Sommer, D. C. Haspinger, M. Andrä, M. Sacherer, C. Viertler, P. Regitnig, and G. A. Holzapfel. Quantification of Shear Deformations and Corresponding Stresses in the Biaxially Tested Human Myocardium. *Annals of Biomedical Engineering*, 43(10):2334–2348, 2015. ISSN 15739686. doi: 10.1007/s10439-015-1281-z.

[81] G. Sommer, A. J. Schriefl, M. Andrä, M. Sacherer, C. Viertler, H. Wolinski, and G. A. Holzapfel. Biomechanical properties and microstructure of human ventricular myocardium. *Acta Biomaterialia*, 24:172–192, 2015. ISSN 18787568. doi: 10.1016/j.actbio.2015.06.031.

[82] H. M. Spotnitz, W. D. Spotnitz, T. S. Cottrell, D. Spiro, and E. H. Sonnenblick. Cellular basis for volume related wall thickness changes in the rat left ventricle. *Journal of Molecular and Cellular Cardiology*, 6(4):317–322, aug 1974. ISSN 0022-2828. doi: 10.1016/0022-2828(74)90074-1.

[83] D. D. Streeter, H. M. Spotnitz, D. P. Patel, J. Ross, and E. H. Sonnenblick. Fiber Orientation in the Canine Left Ventricle during Diastole and Systole. *Circulation Research*, 24(3):339 LP –347, mar 1969. URL `http://circres.ahajournals.org/content/24/3/339.abstract`.

[84] F. A. Syomin and A. K. Tsaturyan. A simple model of cardiac muscle for multiscale simulation: Passive mechanics, crossbridge kinetics and calcium regulation. *Journal of Theoretical Biology*, 420(August 2016):105–116, 2017. ISSN 10958541. doi: 10.1016/j.jtbi.2017.02.021.

[85] N. Thurieau, J.-P. Jehl, R. K. Njiwa, N. Tran, and P. Maureira. Modeling Heart Tissue As a Micromorphic Medium: a Numerical Investigation. *Journal of Mechanics in Medicine and Biology*, 17(05):1750078, 2017. ISSN 0219-5194. doi: 10.1142/S0219519417500786.

[86] S. W. J. Ubbink, P. H. M. Bovendeerd, T. Delhaas, T. Arts, and F. N. van de Vosse. Towards model-based analysis of cardiac MR tagging data: Relation between left ventricular shear strain and myofiber orientation. *Medical Image Analysis*, 10(4):632–641, 2006. ISSN 13618415. doi: 10.1016/j.media.2006.04.001.

[87] T. P. Usyk, R. Mazhari, and A. D. Mcculloch. Effect of Laminar Orthotropic Myofiber Architecture on Regional Stress and Strain in the Canine Left Ventricle. *Journal of elasticity and the physical science of solids*, 61:143–164, 2000.

[88] T. P. Usyk, I. J. LeGrice, and A. D. McCulloch. Computational model of three-dimensional cardiac electromechanics. *Computing and Visualization in Science*, 4(4):249–257, 2002. ISSN 14330369. doi: 10.1007/s00791-002-0081-9.

[89] M. von Hoegen, S. Skatulla, and J. Schroeder. A micromorphic continuum formulation for cardiac tissue mechanics. In *Proceedings of the VI International Conference on Structural Engineering, Mechanics and Computation*, number 1987, 2016. ISBN 9781138029279.

[90] M. von Hoegen, S. Skatulla, and J. Schröder. A generalized micromorphic approach accounting for variation and dispersion of preferred material directions. *Computers and Structures*, 2017. ISSN 00457949. doi: 10.1016/j.compstruc.2017.11.013.

[91] X. Wang and J. D. Lee. Micromorphic theory: A gateway to nano world. *International Journal of Smart and Nano Materials*, 1(2):115–135, 2010. ISSN 19475411. doi: 10.1080/19475411.2010.484207.

[92] J. Wilber and J. Walton. The convexity properties of a class of constitutive models for biological soft issues. *Mathematics and Mechanics of Solids*, 7(3):217, 2002. ISSN 10812865. doi: 10.1177/108128602027726.

[93] J. Wong and E. Kuhl. Generating fibre orientation maps in human heart models using Poisson interpolation, 2014. ISSN 1025-5842.

[94] P. Wriggers. *Nonlinear Finite Element Methods*. Springer, 2008. ISBN 978-3-540-71000-4. doi: 10.1007/978-3-540-71001-1.

[95] Wye River Upper School. Anatomy Physiology - The Heart., 2011. URL `http://www.wyeriverupperschool.org/houserwrus/AnatomyPhysiology/May52011/index.html`.

[96] F. C. Yin, C. C. Chan, and R. M. Judd. Compressibility of perfused passive myocardium. *American Journal of Physiology-Heart and Circulatory Physiology*, 271(5):H1864–H1870, 1996. doi: 10.1152/ajpheart.1996.271.5.H1864.

[97] X. Zeng, Y. Chen, and J. D. Lee. Determining material constants in nonlocal micromorphic theory through phonon dispersion relations. *International Journal of Engineering Science*, 44 (18-19):1334–1345, 2006. ISSN 00207225. doi: 10.1016/j.ijengsci.2006.08.002.

www.ingramcontent.com/pod-product-compliance
Lightning Source LLC
LaVergne TN
LVHW041127150826
845673LV00007B/2204

* 9 7 8 3 3 8 4 2 3 1 1 3 0 *